# SURVIVING MORTALITY

# Surviving Mortality

*Life, Death, and the Doctor*

by

## Roger C. Dunham, M.D.

©2017

ISBN-13:
978-0692977385 (Roger C. Dunham, M.D.)

ISBN-10:
0692977384

# CONTENTS

# PROLOGUE

The patients in this book are real people, and most of them have died.

These are the people who have battled forces driving them into their own unique circumstances of mortality...they have traveled down their individual pathways of life, from their births to their deaths, and most of them have moved—sometimes slowly, sometimes suddenly—into that vast arena of uncertainty often defined in polite post-mortem conversation as the "hereafter." As those of us left behind search for the meaning about this mystery when life is no more, we struggle to comprehend the incomprehensible nature of mortality. We search for answers from the doctor in charge, from the priest, minister, or rabbi at the bedside, from the relatives who have shared the patient's life and suffering. We search within ourselves.

And the answers do not come easily.

There are few words in the English language that have generated so much fascination to the people of our society as "mortality," and few that have increased so much in written usage during the past 200 years. For such a simple word, it is rich with complexity; the concept of mortality stimulates a myriad of meanings. Most of us think of mortality as the end of life—a person lives, and then for innumerable reasons, that person will die. Since each of us is mortal, the inevitable end will always eventually arrive *and it is always final.* However, it is not so simple.

Merriam-Webster struggles to cover all the bases with their comprehensive definition:

Mortality is:

1. *the quality or state of being a person or thing that is alive and therefore certain to die: the quality or state of being mortal*
2. *the death of a person, animal, etc.*
3. *the number of deaths that occur in a particular time or place*

Mortality is, then, formally defined by Merriam-Webster as: alive but with death coming, or perhaps it is the actual death, or if those definitions don't satisfy, it is the number of deaths in a specific setting. The term "death" is more easily understood—it is the absolute **end of life** without return to a viable state, notwithstanding those who like to say this or that person "experienced death but then came back to life." Death means the permanent ending of vital processes in living cells or tissue, *permanent, not reversible.*

That takes care of death, but mortality is something else entirely.

It can all be so confusing, unless you turn to religion. Under the umbrella of understanding within virtually every religion in the world, the "end" is actually the beginning—an individual's mortality and subsequent death is the start of the after-life, or a reincarnation recycled life, the initiation of the hereafter and all that it may represent for those who believe. This takes faith, lots of faith, about what is awaiting us all. And this is a serious matter, for eternity is a very long time: at the mortal moment, the moment of death and following the judgment process, there will be either eternal heaven or eternal hell as the payment for having lived a good life or a bad life.  Or perhaps there will be 72 virgins[1] prepared and waiting to bring sexual pleasure (worth thinking about if the departed is male and less than about 100 years old; it is challenging to determine the reward for a departing female in this context).  Finally, as described in Hinduism, and then Buddhism, there may be a process of reincarnation with a chance to start over again, creating a painful and endless cycle of births and deaths (from which one would hope to escape by entering the abstract state of *nirvana*).

This mortality business is such a challenge. After 40 years of working for my patients in the huge medical spectrum encompassed by the field of Internal Medicine, from the churning intensities at the UCLA School of Medicine, through the dark corridors at the USC/LA County Medical Center, from the homes of distressed patients to the intensive care units of our local hospitals, I have seen almost all that mortality encompasses, *during the time when life still exists*.  I have actively participated in the mortality processes for many of my patients, I have battled to leave the promise of impending mortality unfulfilled for most of my patients, and I have learned along the way that each case, each patient, and each circumstance of suffering is different from the others.  There is no common element that allows a collective consensus about the proper way to manage mortality.  The patients may share certain diagnoses, they may be of similar ages or race, they may have had similar magnitudes of wealth or poverty or positions of importance but they are nowhere close to being the same.

People die in a manner that reflects their unique differences as individual human beings.

And so, when life is over and done, when the last shuddering breath has expired and no movements occur thereafter, the transition from impending mortality into the reality of death arrives. For those with faith, the patient has moved from living into the afterlife or a recycled life. However, the hereafter of each patient is naturally not evident to those of us at the bedside, and words of religion (while soothing to those left behind) do not visibly affect the body on the bed. This is especially true since the soul that is the centerpiece of virtually all religion is beyond our direct observation. The expired patient, with a physical destiny to be buried or to be cremated, will never move again and is not affected by any spoken word from observers of the event. It is at that point where the reality of mortality is fulfilled; in those quick seconds when blood pressure drops to zero and is no more, when the final "expiration" is completed and breathing and thinking are finished, when the "bright light" that some have described at the edge of the precipice has shined and possibly extinguished, that is the point where all of us must ask what was the quality of this mortality process leading to this death?

It is an important question since it only happens once in our lifetime.

We have heard many words to describe this moment, from the patient has "lived a good life," or he died on his motorcycle "doing what he always loved to do," or perhaps "she went peacefully, she didn't linger, she is no longer suffering," or finally, "she is gone now, leaving behind these wonderful children and wonderful grandchildren." Sometimes, I have heard a relative say in that moment of grief, "Well, at least he had a good death," and I have agreed, having seen so many that went badly. The words to define this mortality, then, actually describe the life of the patient prior to death, often the *dying process*, rather than the death *per se*. These words, spoken by the anguished left behind, are words that often define the time *before* that final instant, a statement about the quality found during life, before the dimming and extinguishment of the final gathering of living cells. Since we understand that death itself, the fulfillment of mortality, is irreversible and mysterious, all reflection is about the mortal process itself that precedes death, and that time that ranges from a lifetime of hopeful living to the final moments of death that defines mortality fulfillment.

And so this book, then, is about survival in the face of mortality. From the bedside in the hospital or at home, from the myriad of interventions along the journey to the final moment, this book gives guidance to define a movement away from the rigid recommendations described in so much literature today. SURVIVING MORTALITY addresses the *variance* of mortality, the spectrum determined by each patient's individual circumstances. Fortunately for all of us, many of the circumstances that seem to control our lives, especially those that may accelerate the arrival of mortality, can be changed to improve the pathway to this end — a means to surviving this destiny by knowing the confidential and intimate stories of the patients who have reached their final seconds on this earth.

And with that knowledge, as it applies to the days, years or decades before the last breath, it is indeed possible for all of us to survive mortality.

# CHAPTER 1
## Who Ya Gonna Call?

The call for help came into my home at 3:14 AM, the harsh brain-rattling buzzing noise of the telephone waking me and my wife from deep sleep. For a doctor, it is ominous to receive a call at that early hour and whoever is on the other end is always filled with bad news. Usually, it is the emergency room, and the conversation generally starts with a female voice responding to my sleepy, "Dr. Dunham here."

The usual Emergency Room mechanical voice from the coordinator of the hospital's entry point would say, "Cottage ER here, please hold for Dr. Bartlein."[2]

And then the line would usually be placed on hold, while I would lay there in the dark for sometimes a minute or two, sometimes more, wondering which patient had suffered such circumstances to violate my directions to *always call me first before going to the emergency room.* Perhaps it was a car wreck, perhaps it was a sudden heart attack, something bad and something quick, something to require an ambulance and emergency room care, something that did not allow time for the requested call. Over the years and blessed with attentive patients, I have found that they rarely go to the emergency room voluntarily without contacting me first, and sometimes they would even call *from the paramedic ambulance*, hollering over the noise of the siren.

But this was a different call, there was no delay, no emergency room beeping sounds in the background, and my telephone greeting was immediately answered by a calm female voice, saying, "Roger?"

My patients often call me by my first name, especially those I've been caring for over many years. "Yes, may I help you?"

Beside me, my wife stirred as I talked.

"Thank you, Roger, this is Marianne…."

Marianne Jackson…. My mind raced to her circumstances. A 35-year-old lady, Marianne was definitely my patient, but I knew she was not calling about herself.

"Marianne, what's going on?" I asked, wide awake now.

It was a call about her father, that kind and gentle man who, as a retired family practice and emergency room physician, had led me down his path for the past seven years as he fought the not-so-rare disease known as ALS (amyotrophic lateral sclerosis) or Lou Gehrig's disease. Unlike the most famous patient with the disease, Dr. Stephen Hawkins, this patient's condition had followed the usual progressively downward course in a much shorter period of time of about seven years, his muscles weakening and becoming atrophic, his ability to walk increasingly unstable and finally terminating, his ability to even breathe becoming difficult in spite of everything that could be done by the best neurologists at UCLA, UC San Francisco, or in Santa Barbara. And over those years as the disease progressed and as he had visited my office so many times, his mind stayed sharp and clear, forcing him to continuously bear witness to the daily micro-tragedies of his worsening condition. As a physician, he knew the pattern of progression and he knew the outcome.

"It's my dad..." Marianne's voice choked over the telephone, "I'm sorry to call you at this hour, Roger, but my Dad.... He doesn't seem to be moving. Could you come over and check on him?"

Marianne *never* called me in the middle of the night to check on herself or her mother, or even her father—this was without question a true emergency. She and her mother needed me at her home, right now or as soon as possible. Fortunately enough, what she had not heard when she had called my direct number (all of my patients have my direct number) was the curse of all medical telephone messages in this country, a message repeated by a mechanical recorded voice across the United States, thousands of times each night, *"If this is an emergency, hang up and call 911."*

"I'm on my way," I answered into the telephone. Fifteen minutes later, I arrived at Marianne's father's house. The streets were deserted and dark, but I knew exactly where they lived, in a hilltop view home behind the city. I had been there before...multiple times.

I found Dr. Jackson sitting in his favorite living room chair looking out through his expansive view window at the dark Pacific Ocean and the lights of Santa Barbara. As Marianne had said, he wasn't moving and he showed no response as I crossed the room. His eyes were open and he appeared to be quite comfortable, sitting in a partly reclined position, his stick-thin arms resting on the sides of the chair, his feet propped up on the soft Ottoman before him. His face was thin from having lost nearly a hundred pounds during the past couple of years. He had been taking his supplemental nutrition, and recently had been spoon-fed by Mrs. Jackson and Marianne.

Dr. Peter Jackson was quite dead, of that I was immediately certain. As Marianne and her mother watched, silent and wide-eyed across the room, I quietly performed the ritual that had been my unfortunate burden in these circumstances over the years of my private practice.

I placed my hand on his bony shoulder and I called out, "Peter? Can you hear me?"

When there was no movement and no response, I checked his pupils with my penlight for any response to light. There was no reflexive contraction to the bright light, the pupils were fixed and slightly dilated. Continuing the ritual, I pulled out my blood pressure cuff and wrapped it tightly around his pathologically skinny right biceps. It was like a child's arm, it was so thin, and as I pumped the cuff and watched the pressure meter, I listened for the brachial artery that should begin pulsating its message of life as the cuff relaxed—there was nothing. I unwrapped the cuff and carefully placed the diaphragm of my stethoscope against the protruding ribs of his chest, listening for anything that suggested a beating heart.

4

His chest was as silent as his home on the hill above the night-lights of Santa Barbara.

I put the stethoscope back into my black bag, I gently closed Dr. Jackson's eyes, and I quietly moved to the two women who knew the news before I even spoke a word.

"He is finally at peace, I'm sorry I could not do more."

I gave them a hug, I said some more words, and that was the final moment of Dr. Jackson's mortality, a seven year downhill ride upon an increasingly difficult road, finally ending with my 4 AM call to the soft-speaking mortician to come and gently do his job.

During the time before his death, the patient had not really been "fighting his disease," since there is so little that can be done for that condition beyond support of the systems in his body that are still working. Providing primary care was therefore far beyond the science of medicine and the immediate medical challenges of incurable disease. The examinations over the years, the talks with the patient, the discussions with his wife and with Marianne, the arranging of Visiting Nurse care and finally hospice care, the house calls as needed, with the continuing process of making adjustments for the debilities as they arose. And this defines the needs for just a single patient and his family; at the same time, there are thousands of other patients in most Internal Medicine, Family Practice, and Pediatric practices, each with his or her unique demands and needs.

This is primary care medicine, and this is disappearing from the United States.

The information on this matter is not just alarming, it is shocking with the data confirming this centerpiece of our health care system is vanishing. In one of the more recent studies by the Association of American Medical Colleges (AAMC)[3], the demand for physicians is clearly growing far faster than the supply can provide. And since the total physician demand will increase by nearly 20% between now and 2025, mostly accounted for by the growing and aging population, the forecasted supply of primary care doctors will be more than 20,000 primary care physicians short in the next ten years.

This shortfall is unprecedented, and although statistics tend to blur the mind, when you look at Marianne's challenges, and when you think of the circumstances of a single family with a single illness and a single urgent need in the early hours of the morning, the consequences of this shortage become evident.

Furthermore, this is not just a problem for the elderly, it is a problem for our entire population. After a quick glance at our threatened Medicare system, our threatened Social Security System, and now the primary care physician shortage, the question that needs to be answered is, where are all these patients coming from and why are there not enough doctors?

The increasing life expectancy of patients in the United States, an astounding 30 year increase (from 47 years to nearly 80 years since 1900, largely from better health care, vaccinations, and reduced infant mortality) accounts for much of the senior population increase. This past year, however, as the result of opioid-related deaths in the United States, life expectancy had decreased by 0.1 years since 2015, to 78.6 years.[4] The final life expectancy data is furthermore affected by ever-increasing new patient immigration from foreign countries and by the surge of "Baby-Boomers," those post-war babies now reaching 55-70 years of age.

On the other side of the spectrum is the diminishing supply of physicians and the inadequate number of new primary care doctors. Among my physician colleagues across the United States, an interesting question is, what is your son or daughter going to be when he or she grows up? Contrary to the past, these young people (who have seen up-close the lives of their doctor-parent) are opting for *any* career other than medicine. Everywhere, from those who report on this subject, we hear "it is the low pay" preventing premedical and medical students from moving into primary care, or from even becoming *any* kind of doctor. While the pay for the rigorous years of training (at ever-increasing great expense) for primary care doctors is near the bottom of the physician pay scale, this is not the primary reason for the shortage. Simply stated, doctors in active practice across the United States are unhappy with their day-to-day lives and it is getting worse. And since one in three doctors is currently over the age of 50 (most doctors don't even start their practices of medicine until about the age of 30 because of the long training time), and since most primary care physicians are now wanting to retire sooner rather than later, the shortage is rapidly worsening. Furthermore, every time a doctor hangs up his or her stethoscope, the patients of that practice must find a new doctor—and those doctors are then becoming forced to examine more and more patients each hour, resulting in worsening care, worsening access, and greater dissatisfaction.

Amazingly, it is even much worse than that....

As these aging doctors are dragged into the computer world, there was...briefly...the hope that streamlining of data acquisition would improve the delivery of care. Not surprisingly, this computerization of data has led instead to an onerous intrusion into private medical practices by bean-counter payment systems, both public and private. How intrusive can this get? In just the past couple of years, it was announced that the Federal Government would pay physicians if they conduct discussions with patients about "end-of-life" care, such as how patients may have their lives ended *early* by the physicians or by themselves, bringing an obvious cost-savings to the Medicare budget by their deaths. Is this possible, I ask? How can the government decide to pay doctors to conduct this or that specific discussion in the private setting of a doctor's office? And these discussions, determined by bureaucrats without MD degrees, will be monitored for their, what? For their political correctness? For their cost-savings benefit? Furthermore, the discussion of other items will *not* be met with reimbursement? What about discussions relating to giving medicine to provide comfort, or medicines that might allow a longer life? Discussions about the cardiac angina or about the tremor? Is that allowed? Will the government pay for that? At what point will the doctor be inclined to throw his or her stethoscope into the dumpster and ask the Spirit of Hippocrates whatever in the world has happened to the essence of Medicine?

But the government and the insurance companies say that all a doctor has to do is properly code for the service provided. Code right and payment will come. But, as individual doctors try to apply computer codes that accurately reflect the care provided, they are facing entire buildings filled with computers designed to NOT pay for provided care because of every imaginable reason...the list for non-payment is endless. In the middle of all this, emerging like a Frankenstein of Medicine, is the latest payment system to be used by the government and enthusiastically embraced by the private insurance industry: ICD-10. This monster is the 10th revision of the International Statistical Classification of Diseases and Related Health Problems (ICD), a medical classification list by the World Health Organization (WHO). The adoption of this creature by the "CMS" (Centers for Medicare and Medicaid Services), following the WHO, is a perfect example of this non-payment problem. Packing ICD-10 into doctors' computers creates a nightmare of labyrinthine proportions, implemented every day with every keystroke by the government, Blue Cross and everyone else, to theoretically allow or block reimbursement for doctors, without significant modification or oversight by our elected representatives or the people of our country.

The tortuous pathway of this system's development underscores the virtually futile effort to categorize every element of human experience for the purpose of reimbursement—it reads like a saga of bureaucratic exuberance. All of this system's mandates are for the purpose of refusing reimbursement, *and never for the purpose of improving health care.* Originally mandated in 1999, the ICD-10 deadline for adoption "for reimbursement" of physician care was then changed to 2009, then 2011, then in October 2013. Then, a *deadline of 2014 was set, and more recently, the deadline was set at* October 1, 2015. In this system, doctors looking to send a bill for their services must become aware of the following guidelines: The basic structure is clarified as: Characters 1-3 (the category of disease); 4 (etiology of disease); 5 (body part affected), 6 (severity of illness) and 7 (placeholder for extension of the code to increase specificity). Not only must new software be installed and tested in each doctor's computer, but also medical practices must provide training for physicians, staff members, and administrators and will need to develop new practice policies and guidelines, and update paperwork and forms.

Moving from the 14,000 diagnoses found in ICD-9 to the 70,000+ diagnoses in ICD-10, the diagnoses now includes not just time spent with a patient, but such diagnoses as, "Struck by a duck," "Sucked into a Jet Engine," "Bizarre personal appearance," "Accident while Knitting or Crocheting," and "Burn due to water-skis on fire." At the time of this writing, there is no code for "Hit by a Drone," but I understand it is coming. This is an actual system, required for billing purposes by the insurance companies and the government entitlement systems. If nothing else this has become a remarkably efficient system to ensure that these "payers" will not pay. And when the primary care doctor is not paid, or his or her payment is significantly reduced or delayed (as it almost always is), the challenge leads to the doctor's immediate problem of covering the approximately 40% of overhead costs just for billing staff (with minimum wage requirements, insurance requirements, sick day requirements, training requirements, taxation mandates, liability protection, workman's comp expenses, etc.) and equipment *solely to figure out what code should be used in the billing*. Importantly, this is not to improve care and this is not to allow more time from the doctor to provide care; this does nothing to allow doctors to make house calls at 3:30 in the morning or to see patients in the emergency room.

If there ever was an orchard of "Family Trees of Doctors," it now seems to be withering and dying off as very few bright young children can now look to his or her physician father or mother and see satisfaction with the profession. The consequences of all this are that shortages get worse, foreign-trained physicians, nurse practitioners, and Physician Assistants with two years of training beyond college are increasingly being inserted in the place of doctors while individual physicians are forced to see more and more patients, accelerating physician burn-out and early retirement.

If we are facing a shortage of tens of thousands of primary care physicians right now, and it takes around ten years to produce new doctors, how many calls like Marianne's will go unanswered, or at the very least will result in greatly added expense to individuals and to the tax-paying public? Take a *single case* of a daughter who needs help because her father is approaching the end of his life and now doesn't seem to be moving much, and ask who is going to take the call when there is no primary care doctor available?

Should she call a national "Doctors-On-Call Virtual Care" line? Does she call 911? And when the operator asks, "What is the nature of your emergency?" must she say that her dad has been sick but is trying to survive.... "Is this an emergency?" the operator may ask, or "What are his symptoms?" Should an ambulance be sent, should there be red lights and sirens at 3 AM through the darkened streets of Santa Barbara? Is he hauled away on a cold gurney into the paramedic van? Does he need to be in the emergency room, mixed with the hordes of beleaguered patients who are seeking their own diagnoses, does he need a doctor to declare him to have expired, is he dead, do you think?

Increasingly, the question now should be why anybody with a brain and powers of observation would ever decide that entering the field of primary care medicine would be a good idea?

But, why not throw the moneychangers out of the primary care Temple of Medicine?

If this happens, as the Medicare, Medicaid, and insurance company billing systems disappear, they will be followed out the doctor's door by ICD-10 software and the billing clerks that are clogging the rooms of the offices, and consuming so much money. And what is left? Just the patient and the doctor, each able to work together without the dark elements of control from bureaucrats and others who know nothing about medicine. The patient, while keeping a relatively inexpensive "catastrophic" or high-deductible policy, becomes free to choose a doctor without having to announce he or she is "a Medicare patient," or under this or that insurance plan, since none of this really matters any more. And the doctor becomes free to provide care based on patients' needs, not based on what ICD-10 and the computer gurus in distant cities might allow. Just by completely quitting Medicare, the doctor can suddenly return to the practice of medicine, caring for Medicare and all other patients *outside the payment system.*

A return to the real "fee for service" or to payments made annually or monthly by patients wanting the best of primary care is a return to the practice of medicine without the burden of a system that is devouring medicine. And with less time spent on billing (especially with annual or semi-annual payments, the so-called concierge model), the care and the time available for care greatly increases while the patients may continue to use Medicare and the insurance systems to cover the costs of expensive surgery or hospitalizations. Also, the patients will increasingly elect the available "catastrophic care" insurance plans with vastly reduced premium payments. Finally, and helping reduce the cost of health care in our country, ambulance needs and hospitalizations costs go down since decent *preventive* primary care becomes more available to lower the incidence of diabetes, hypertension, and many other preventable diseases that lead to expensive care.

With this, the practice of medicine becomes pure, and as all communications from Medicare or the insurance companies are thrust into the shredding machines, primary care practices may return to the days gone by even though payments from grateful patients may occasionally be nothing much more than a chicken. Also, with this, the children of medical families might again want to become doctors, more medical students will look longingly at primary care as an endpoint, and the future Marianne families of our country may see the return of house calls to help in their time of need.

The result would be that we will have a happier and healthier country, and when the daughter of the next Dr. Jackson calls for help, the telephone will be answered and help will be promptly provided...like in the "old days."

# CHAPTER 2
## Fulminant Fury or Gentle Guidance

One of the great challenges of practicing medicine is having a front-row seat with an *up close* witnessing of some of the most powerful forces of nature. Watching them or participating in them is not for the timid. And while observing or helping with, for example, the birth of a baby may be an intense process that is usually exciting and occasionally terrifying, there is a pretty clear picture in everybody's mind as what will be happening with the baby after the process is complete. The newborn infant will be placed on the mother's chest, or after pictures are taken and everybody exchanges congratulations, a swathing will occur and the baby will take a nap in the bassinette.

On the other hand, a human being's mortality is almost always chilling because, right up to that very last instant of life, and beyond that time, there is uncertainty about what happens to the star of the show after death. And so, this event with such irreversible results, whether ushered in as a vicious powerhouse of nature that removes victims from this world with thunder and without remorse, or an ironically gentle process that leads the patient toward the same fulfillment of his or her mortality with a quiet peacefulness, it is always riveting at the end and almost always filled with questions that are difficult to answer.

The final picture and the final answers often are found in the hospital basement morgue where a diligent pathologist quietly searches for clues lying within the body of the recently departed.

The reality of these forces came to me early while I was still in my Internal Medicine training program. No longer a medical student or a lowly intern, I was now a "resident" doctor (still in training, not yet certified in anything), returning to the emergency room rotation after a pleasant lunch in the doctors' dining room in an excellent Pasadena hospital named Huntington Memorial Hospital. I had seen about fifteen patients that morning under the watchful eye of the senior emergency physician, with various ailments such as lacerations, migraine headaches, and aches and pains, all diagnosed and all resolved. The patients had subsequently been sent back to their homes without problem. It had been an interestingly nice morning, people seen, people fixed, people happy and sent home.

As I started to walk into a room holding an elderly man with a fever and cough, a paramedic ambulance came screaming up to the emergency room entrance. Normally, the paramedics turn off their sirens a block or so before reaching the hospital, but in this case, the sirens screamed right up to the emergency room's sliding glass doors—a very bad sign. I left the coughing man and went out to see what was happening. Two paramedics jumped out and raced around to the back doors of the ambulance, quickly pulled a gurney holding a writhing man out of their van and accelerated him into the intensive care area. The patient was quickly identified as a 68-year-old man named Joseph Tomascas; he was covered with blood and, as they thrust him into the high-intensity triage room, he abruptly vomited copious amounts of blood into a steel bowl by his head.

The paramedics, usually models of controlled professionalism, were uncharacteristically passionate.

"Found on the sidewalk, bleeding out of both ends!" the female paramedic hollered as she stepped back to allow our group of nurses, ER doctors, and doctors-in-training (me) to cluster around the distressed patient. The bowl contained a couple of cups of bright red blood, rapidly emptied into a sink by a nurse. The man's jeans were covered with additional expanding stains of blood moving down his legs.

"Blood pressure 95 over 40, pulse 122!" the paramedic hollered as they moved him into one of the intense-care rooms and the nurses began cutting off the man's jeans to gain access to his abdomen. "Two IV's with Ringer's going wide open!" she added as the man yelled, "Don't let me die!" and promptly vomited another cup of blood into the bowl.

"Was he shot or stabbed or what, any available history?" I asked as we slapped cardiac leads onto his arms and ran a catheter into his bladder, returning a thimble of dark yellow urine.

"Negative gunshot or knifing, negative trauma!" the male paramedic called out over the loud beeping of the man's heart from the cardiac monitor system. "Negative alcohol, negative ulcer history, no GI history, no meds except occasional Tylenol! No Coumadin! No allergies! Had Triple A surgery seven years ago, no other surgery!"

Triple A, meaning AAA or Abdominal Aortic Aneurysm, the curse of a bulging aorta in the abdomen, threatening rupture, usually repaired in those days by replacing the enlarged aorta with the insertion of a Dacron graft, hopefully placed into the depths of the abdomen before the aorta ruptures. If the aneurysm begins to rupture before the graft is placed, it quickly fills the abdomen with blood from the leaking aorta and the patient usually experiences a precipitous blood pressure drop with an associated very high probability of dying. However, it generally does not cause the GI tract blood that seemed to cover the gurney.

"Don't let me die!" the man hollered again as I moved my hands around his abdomen, searching for tumors, bulging or tenderness. Except for a midline scar from his previous surgery, his slender abdomen was unremarkable.

A shrill alarm went off on the wall over my head. "Blood Pressure down to 90 systolic, pulse 130!" the nurse hollered. The man vomited blood again and screamed for us to save him as our team completed our high-speed examination. The senior emergency physician ordered six units of blood and medication "pressers" to try and increase his blood pressure as the operating room upstairs called that a room was available when ready. Two surgeons and an anesthesiologist evaluated Tomascas as he vomited more blood, screamed more pleadings for salvation and with severely shaking hands, signed clearance for us to hustle him off to the operating room. It was my job to accompany him up to the third floor in the elevator with a nurse, Marie Dubra, one of the senior emergency room veterans.

With the cardiac monitor on the gurney between Tomascas' legs becoming contaminated with his blood and emitting an incessant cascade of high-speed cardiac beeps, the elevator door closed and Tomascas abruptly became unconscious before the elevator even began to move. Marie frantically tried to measure his blood pressure as the elevator moved up and the beeping of the cardiac monitor accelerated. Before we passed the first floor, the monitor abruptly showed a fibrillating heart and then a flat line, while emitting the continuous nightmarish whine of a heart that had moved into a full cardiac arrest.

By the time the elevator door opened on the surgical floor, I was already on the gurney, on top of the patient, pumping his chest while getting covered with his blood as the anesthesiologist quickly rushed up and inserted a tube into his windpipe to deliver 100% oxygen under direct pressure to his lungs. I continued to compress his chest, we did everything I had ever been taught to perform an effective Code Blue procedure, we injected his heart directly with adrenaline and we shocked him with the chest paddles numerous times. We squeezed the IV bags to deliver more fluid into his veins, more blood flowed out onto the gurney; he never regained consciousness or a heartbeat. Finally, after forty-five minutes of doing everything possible, I decided it was to no avail.

I declared Mr. Tomascas dead at 1:15 PM, right outside the operating room doors.

Standing back from the man's gurney, blood still running off my green scrubs and blood dripping on the floor off the dead man's arm still draped over the side, I felt like I had just witnessed a gigantic train of death *carrying one passenger* who was screaming for help as he accelerated down the tracks of life and off the end of the rails to his total and final oblivion. All I could see that anybody had been able to do for poor Tomascas from the moment the paramedics picked him up to the end of his life was to *very slightly* delay the moment of his actual death.

Later that afternoon, the hospital pathologist called me to advise that the aorta and the graft of Tomascas had started leaking and had pulsated a hole into his small intestine, creating a pathway for blood, a so-called "fistula" or aberrant pathway carrying aorta blood straight into his intestinal track. It was an unpredictable kind of thing, the pathologist had said, and since nobody had known about the impending disaster, and nobody had therefore operated on the man an hour or more *before* symptoms of the bleeding became evident, the fistula that threw him unto the train of death was his final coup de grace, delivered by the powerful fist of nature.

Obviously, Mr. Tomascas did not die a good death. It was sudden but it was truly a terrible way to move into his hereafter, like a man shot by a huge gun from nature, leaving him bleeding and hollering, "Don't let me die! Don't let me die!" But to this young doctor still in residency training, still trying to develop confidence that acts of nature might be resolved or prevented by well-educated and well-considered acts of medicine, this was raw education that emphasizes the need for those of us in our profession to recognize the power of what is actually lurking out there. And as

I spent the next half hour in the emergency room shower, intensely scrubbing Mr. Tomascas' blood from every part of my body, the evidence was right there before me…no matter what was done, no matter how much I had learned during the years before or how hard I had worked to save him, and no matter how badly I did not want it to happen, the man died, he died terribly. And there was virtually nothing I could do about it.

I came out of the shower feeling about ten years older than when I had started the emergency room shift that morning.

Almost as sudden, but in sharp contrast to Tomascas, was Mr. Stephen Bartholomew, the man with bad knees who came to me for care several years later, long after I completed my training and became a board certified Internal Medicine physician. At 77 years of age, lean and tough, Bartholomew was very smart, very wealthy, and a perfect example of a patient with ragingly good health—almost a poster-child of how great we can all be if we take good care of ourselves. Living in a mansion of a home in the hills of Santa Barbara with his loving wife, he had developed his international business to the point where money was never going to be an issue, even if he lived another hundred years…Bartholomew was tough and seemed nearly *impervious* to anything nature might bring his way.

But his vigorous daily exercise program had worn down the cartilage in his knees, bone-on-bone, and the pain had become an annoyance in his daily life. He came to me for help, I found him an excellent orthopedic surgeon, I screened the man with treadmills and a thorough pre-op medical exam, and on a sunny Wednesday afternoon, Bartholomew underwent orthopedic surgery to replace his left knee. The surgery was successful, the surgeon called his wife and then he called me to announce the excellent outcome. At 7 PM, I stopped by his hospital room to make sure all was well.

"No problems," his nurse, an attractive young lady who liked to be called "Missy," informed me as she accompanied me into the room.

"No problems!" Mr. Bartholomew immediately roared to both of us, adding with a smile, "That was so easy, Doc, I'm going to get my *other* knee replaced in a month!"

I said something appropriate, like, "When you are as healthy as you are, life is good!" and we left the room.

He was clearly a decisive man of action, his wife visited him for a couple of hours and, equally happy with his surgical outcome, she left the hospital at about 9:30 PM.

At 11:30, Missy called my home phone to inform me that Mr. Bartholomew was dead.

"*What*?" I hollered into the telephone. "*Dead? What happened?*"

"I don't know what happened, Dr. Dunham," Missy said, sounding like she was struggling to control her emotions. "I honest-to-God don't know. I went into the room to check on him around 10:30 and I thought he was asleep. He never needed a monitor, since he was doing so well, so there was nothing to indicate there was any problem. But he didn't answer me. I couldn't awaken him, I couldn't get a blood pressure, I called a full code-blue, we worked on him for almost an hour, and all he showed was complete cardiac arrest, his heart never twitched a heartbeat, he was absolutely unresponsive."

"Jesus holy Christ," I muttered under my breath. "Does his wife know about this?"

There was a pause, and then Missy answered in a very tiny voice, "I thought you might want to do that. I'm getting ready to call the surgeon."

After two minutes of concentrated thinking, I called Mrs. Bartholomew to gently break the bad news. An answering machine recording came into my ear. There are some messages I will never leave on answering machines and this was right at the top of the list. I slammed the phone down and I called again. Same answering machine. I left a message for Mrs. Bartholomew to call me ASAP, I put away the small glass of wine I had been enjoying, and I waited. And I waited and I waited. By 1 AM, nobody had called. By 2 AM, I slowly dozed off in the chair and finally went to sleep.

At 2:47 AM, Mrs. Bartholomew called me, and before the phone even reached my ear, I could hear her voice screaming out of the earpiece, "DR. DUNHAM, IS THIS SOME KIND OF TERRIBLE JOKE?????"

Mrs. Bartholomew had left the hospital and visited friends late into the night; after arriving home, she had gone to sleep without checking her telephone. What happened next fulfilled a medical variant of Murphy's Law[5] that says "Anything that can possibly go wrong, does, and when it does go wrong, it will go wrong at the worst possible time, and it will cause the greatest possible damage."

At 2:45 AM, she had been awakened by a national transplant agency, a soft-spoken man had apologized for the early morning call, and confirmed that he was speaking to Mr. Bartholomew's next-of-kin.

"You are talking with Mrs. Bartholomew," she had answered curtly as she awakened. "And what is your name again?"

He then identified himself and asked if she could kindly give verbal authorization in their recorded conversation for the transplanting "into needy patients" her husband's corneas from his eyes, his liver, his heart, his kidneys, and anything else…before she screamed, she hung up the telephone and speed-dialed me.

Ten seconds after I finished that call, I had a horrified and outraged Nurse Missy on the hospital telephone screaming to me, "I *told* them, I *absolutely told* them not to call Mrs. Bartholomew until the doctor had talked with her. Those *idiots*!!!"

And so, after contacting the mortified orthopedic surgeon, I found myself in the dark of the early morning hours sitting on a couch in the living room of a mansion in the hills above Santa Barbara, quietly explaining the unexplainable to the widow of the recently deceased Mr. Bartholomew.

The next morning, the pathologist called me to advise that the autopsy was without abnormalities and that Mr. Bartholomew was an absolutely normal human being. Normal, he added, except for an artificial left knee and his being dead. His heart, his brain, his lungs, his kidneys…he went on and on covering everything known to medicine, all was remarkably normal. And he confirmed that no part of

24

the patient had been sent anywhere except to various bottles in the pathology department.

"Well, that's great but the man is dead," I observed quietly. "There is a reason, there has to be a reason. Please do something else, intensify the investigation, do some microscopic examinations, do some toxin tests, do anything you can think of. We need an answer beyond just thinking that his time has come."

The pathologist called me back the next day with the results of his much more detailed exam. A microscopic examination of Bartholomew's cardiac electrical conducting system had discovered the presence of significant amyloid, a thick waxy abnormal protein material that can rapidly build up in people's bodies over the years, or in Mr. Bartholomew's case, in his heart, as a part of his unidentified and incurable disease, amyloidosis. There is no reliable test for this disease. The amyloid had created a sudden complete heart block during his post-operative state, rendering him unconscious almost immediately as his heart had stopped. Lying there with his brand new knee in place, snuggled under his clean sheets and warm blanket, he had been comfortable in his hospital bed. A few seconds later, Mr. Bartholomew became very quickly, very peacefully, and very permanently dead.

Two different deaths, both of them sudden and unexpected, and neither Tomascas nor Bartholomew had a chance to survive their respective departures from the living. If they had been given a choice, we could speculate, the amyloid flipping of the cardiac switch was preferable to the violent flailing in a sea of blood while pleading for salvation; but neither man had a choice. Furthermore, neither man was aware of his own impending mortality during the hours or days before the event in spite of the absolute certainty that mortality would soon descend upon both of them. If Tomascas had had a Living Will, it almost certainly would have said that he would choose the opportunity to die without suffering, to go in peace without pain or the bloody disaster in the elevator. And if Bartholomew's Living Will had been reviewed, asking for the same, it would have been fulfilled as quiet and peaceful *but not so soon, not so unexpected, and not without saying goodbye to his wife or his children*, he would have said. Both men starting their day with perceived futures, both with the belief of a personal destiny far beyond what they experienced, both suddenly slammed by their respective mortality.

And so, it must be asked, if both men **had** known what was going to happen, that they would both be dead within the next few hours *even though they felt perfectly fine at the moment*, what would they say besides, "No, please no, I'm not ready!" The forces of nature would not be listening. The reality for both men, the reality for all of us in the final microseconds of life, is that there is no time left to do what we might have delayed. The famous bucket list implies that we know about when the end is going to come and have plenty of time to live more of life, but so often we don't have a clue. We need to ask ourselves regularly, then, what do we want for this lifetime we are allotted that allows the best life possible? How would we look at our past, at our recent years, at our lovers and our successes or failures, when we may not perceive this mortality that is suddenly (and irrevocably) at our doorstep?  Would we find satisfaction that life has been as fulfilling as possible?  If we knew life would end in the next days or hours, would we be wondering if we had fulfilled our destinies, however that may be perceived by ourselves or others?  What would we have said to our children, what money should we have passed on to charity, what would we have told somebody who had harmed us or somebody who had been kind to us?

This consideration of rapidly approaching mortality was actually debated among the men of my submarine during my years in the Navy under the Pacific Ocean.[6]  We almost sank on a couple of occasions when various near-disasters occurred either with our nuclear reactor or with our piping systems. On a submarine, cruising along hundreds of feet below the surface, when something goes wrong and we sink deeper into the ocean, all of us would think about the consequences of a rapid approach toward the "collapse depth" — that cataclysmic depth of the ocean when pipes rupture, compartments collapse and sudden tremendous seawater pressure ends everybody's life, all pretty much at the same instant.  This is, perhaps, why submariners are bonded so close far more than most others in the military, for when we are asleep while submerged, or eating dinner, or maybe reading a book, we must rely on the other men on watch to do their jobs exactly right, preventing us from suddenly accelerating downward toward that "collapse depth" that the 16,000 foot deep Pacific Ocean held for us.  It was almost like we were hovering above a huge black hole every moment of every day.

We would debate, the men on our boat, if the engine room flooded, if the propulsion failed, if we angled downward toward the distant bottom, soon to reach the inevitable black hole collapse depth, what would we do just before that instant of time? I had a sample of this one day (or night, most of us never cared much since at our depth it didn't matter), when I was in my rack, sound asleep. With no warning, ocean water suddenly roared out of the ventilation outlet next to my head, essentially blowing me out of my bunk to join the twenty or so other men who also were being flooded out of their racks. As the submarine's loudspeakers suddenly blared throughout the ship, "Now, flooding, flooding! Surface, surface, surface!" At that moment, to our collective shock, we all felt the bow of the ship dropping in the wrong direction: *down* toward the collapse depth.

It also quickly dawned on all of us that a *second* horrible thing was simultaneously happening: the sea water was flooding across the decking in the direction of the massive batteries below the deck, soon to create an electrolysis of the salt water threatening that we might suddenly taste the lethal pepper and pineapple taste as we prepared to abruptly *die of chlorine gas poisoning*. My immediate thought at that instant was something close to "Oh, God, NO, NO!!!" similar to Mr. Tomascas screaming in the emergency room. And we all stared at our impending fate with horror, death by gas poisoning or death by collapse depth crushing/drowning? Death by one or the other, maybe both, and nothing any of us could do about it. The terror of the moment, knowing we had maybe a minute, maybe two minutes before the end, gave each of us a chance to recognize what we should do next before the final goodbye occurred.

The speculation among the submarine debaters of the subject during our pre-disaster rambling debates had, on one occasion, concluded that the soon-to-die sailor should seek out whichever crew member had been unpleasant the day before and quickly smack him in the face, a final satisfying payback of sorts. Since the end would come shortly thereafter, it was reasoned, he probably wouldn't have time to smack you back. We had all laughed at that thought, a kind of protective mental effort that said no such horrible event was ever going to happen to any of us.

However, in the few seconds of feeling the bow point down toward the dark collapse depth below, with seawater flooding around me, with impending death from at least two possible events, my primary thought was immense fear that there was *nothing I could do about anything*. It was the helplessness of the moment that created the most fear. The helplessness of the fact that I was probably going to die, very soon, and that I all I could do was just hang on to the edge of the rack for support as the water flooded in around me and other men in the control center worked to get us to the surface. For us, however, nicely enough, we soon began to feel the bow rise abruptly, the air around us became filled with the sounds of the ballast tanks blowing out water to lighten our submarine, the seals above the battery held back the sea water, and we headed at high speed to the surface. Two days later, we reached Pearl Harbor to repair the hydraulics of our bow planes and our submarine's failed snorkel valve.

These events emphasize a reality that is often ignored in our world—that of an acceleration from the morning "that started just like any other day" and ended in the hereafter with a sudden death or a sudden near-death that was not anticipated. We hear repeatedly in our society that we must plan and we must prepare for all the possible endings in our lives. We hear from "long-term care planners" how important it is to have a "plan" that covers the "home" in which we'll possibly spend years withering away. We hear from financial advisors the significance of having money stashed away, to have retirement accounts, to save in tax-deferred accounts, and so on. And, from the government, what do we hear?

From the government, everything is based on tables that describe the timing of mortality. This mortality, it needs to be emphasized, is never for the individual, it is always for the masses, the very essence of statistics. And so the government (and almost everybody else above the age of 40) looks closely at two things:

1. Life expectancy in North America for those born in 2017 is 81 years for females, 79 years for males[7] (now, decreasing because of opioid overdoses).

2. How much money you must withdraw from your IRA or Defined Benefits tax deferred savings accounts (calculated by dividing the amount of money you've saved by what the table calls the "age-specific distribution period")[8] all based on longevity and calculated so that when you finally die, all of your saved money is

taxed…hopefully at a lower level than when you earned it.

All this is fine except that these important facts of life are based on assumptions of mortality and *the assumptions are virtually always wrong.* How many people that you have known in your lifetime will live precisely 81 or 79 years? What has this knowledge done for Tomascas and Bartholomew and how did it affect the 21-year-old submariner? The assumption we all tend to make, as we get older and allow for more regular physical exams, more attention to blood pressure and blood sugar levels, is that if we're careful, we'll all likely live far beyond what the statistics predict—for about half our population this is true.

Trying to determine how long each of us will live is the greatest bet of our lifetime, and there is no way to know with certainty when our final day will arrive.

For all of us, however, it is worthwhile to cover the bet by not just following the advice from a capable doctor or financial advisor but to also break out of any mold that may constrain your activities and have a great deal of fun and adventure along the way. This means that the "bucket list" should not have just a few items, it should be huge, involving challenge and travel, or the creation of something you might otherwise delay, and it should bring great satisfaction for having done so. As we will see in future chapters, it helps to have created a family, it helps to have actually saved some money (although this is not necessary for many bucket-list items), and it helps to avoid the blatantly dangerous activities that ensure mortality headlines in the local newspapers.

Recently, this concept was summarized succinctly by a teenager, Jake Bailey, in New Zealand shortly after being informed of his being terminally ill from a malignancy.[9] "Be great, be gracious," he said in a speech to his high school classmates, "and be grateful for the opportunities that you have. None of us gets out of life alive. Forget about long-term dreams—let's be passionately dedicated to the pursuit of short-term goals," he said to his rapt audience. "We don't know where we might end up or when it might end up."

And so, the message is clear. The end could come at any time, in spite of our best efforts to drive carefully, to see our doctor regularly, and to pay attention to the various clogged artery potentials or cancer potentials. The end may come from diseases with names nobody can pronounce, much less understand. This could happen to any of us at any time, and a blind assumption that all of life will continue on, tomorrow, next month, or next year, could easily be wrong.

This is the lesson of Tomascas and Bartholomew and for the men in the submarines, the lesson from Jake Bailey, and the lesson for everyone who drives cars or flies airplanes or crosses the street in marked crosswalks. This is the lesson that should be near the top of our minds on a daily basis, mixed between all the things we must do to survive, to thrive, and along the way, to find pleasure and meaning, and to have fun as we live our lives.

# CHAPTER 3
## How Old is Too Old?

They called me from the hospital emergency room one afternoon about Mrs. Evelyn Pitsdale, tne ER coordinator telling me a patient had just been brought in by the paramedics and that Dr. Bosner needed to talk with me. Within an amazing ten seconds, he was on the line.

"We have one of your ladies here in the ER, Roger," Bosner told me, "a Mrs. Pitsdale, elderly frail gal on insulin, just blacked-out earlier today."

"That would be Evelyn..." I started.

"Yup, she was with her daughter, shopping downtown, suddenly blacked out, brought in by the paramedics."

My thoughts about this lady raced through my mind. Evelyn Pitsdale, my thin, 95-year-old white-haired patient for the past 15 years who lives at home, prepares her own meals, takes her medications, and somehow manages to give herself exactly the right dose of insulin, injected every day.

"Hypoglycemic?" I asked, jumping to a likely cause of a blackout—an insulin "reaction" from her insulin shot generating an excessively low blood sugar.

"Nope," Bosner said. "That's what we all thought, but her finger-stick glucose was 130 on the site, and she had already awakened when the paramedics arrived."

"How is her heart and her blood pressure?"

This is how the conversations begin, discussing the senior citizens of our community who become sick, the aging people who are delivered to the emergency rooms, often with the words "elderly and frail" at the beginning of the discussion. Implied, but never said, are other words, such as "ready to go, at the end of life, circling the drain, making the final dive." Physicians are involved with this regularly, when mortality decisions arrive in the doctors' daily life, often because of "advanced age." A family member might say, "Look how old he is…. The time has come." Or, "She is really elderly now, she shouldn't continue to suffer." And sometimes patients themselves will say, "I'm just too old to go on, let me go so I can join Papa in the heavens."

Age is naturally one of the most powerful ingredients mixed into the soup of mortality and there is consistently a presumption that older patients are near the end of life, *primarily because they are older.*

What is old and how much does age actually play a role? We know we would do everything possible to save a 7-year-old who, because of accident or disease, is facing his or her mortality. We would do the same for a 35-year-old, or most 50-year-olds. But what about somebody who is 65, or maybe 80? The gray zone of decision-making arrives around 55-60 and then everything starts to become difficult. What about somebody who is 95 years old, like poor Mrs. Pitsdale?

Is she too old to continue?  Where is the line between "We have to save her!" and "The time has come for suffering to end"?  And at what age should we say about ourselves, "My time has come, I am too old to go on…."?

Is there an age out there when it is in fact a time to go?  As far as the government is concerned, the head of the Centers for Medicare and Medicaid Services (CMS) struggles with the financial challenges of Medicare daily; as noted previously, they will now pay for physicians to talk with patients reaching the advanced age of 65 (Medicare age for most people) about ending it all…*and perhaps, from a financial standpoint, (wink, wink) the sooner the better*?  And also, now, the government will finance discussions about an earlier, more convenient, more cost-effective, finale to even *younger* Medicare patients with chronic disabilities.  However, most people are well aware that the government is a terrible source for such profound decisions, (really, "push Grandma's wheelchair off the cliff" because the government encourages the concept?)  The very creepiness of these kinds of state-sponsored death discussions or financial encouragements, brings thoughts of another era, on another continent, where a "Final Solution" from a government source gained credibility, became accepted by the citizens, and underwent implementation with disastrous consequences.  And doesn't this all suggest a grossly inappropriate intrusion of government bureaucrats into private doctor-patient conversations?  Should the government really know what doctors and patients talk about behind the closed doors of our examination rooms, and should the government really offer to pay for specific discussions?

The passing of time that creates the aging process is, of course, the primary accelerant to the final point of mortality that defines the end of life. And yet, while the movement of time and the accumulation of years play such a predominant role with aging, there are many other factors that also may have an effect, often a huge effect, on this process. Some people seem to get old fast for a variety of reasons. We are all intrinsically aware of this variability, and in social gatherings we frequently hear greetings to someone who has not been seen for several years, to someone who looks remarkably older than might be accounted by time. Sometimes the appearance of these individuals can be shocking, but we never exactly hear it stated that way. It is not nice to make such observations. For example, we *never* hear anybody say, "Well, hello, it's been awhile now but, honestly, you are looking so old!" Furthermore, I can't recall hearing at any family gathering or social setting, "*My God*, look at all the wrinkles you've gathered, you are becoming older than sin!" and we never hear such not so thinly-veiled comments like, "What in the holy hell has happened to your face?"

For smokers, the acceleration of aging is a given, recognized by observers everywhere and by most physicians. Furthermore, the 1-2 pack per day smoker does not just *look* older, mostly from a more rapid accumulation of wrinkles, mixed with the "smoker's cough" and the raspy voice, but the smoker actually *is* older (without the accumulation of years) by almost every other signpost of aging. The smoker has accelerated aging factors that include osteoporosis, susceptibility to infection or to most major cancers, frailty and inability to breathe adequately because of "tobacco emphysema," or even blindness, heart disease and stroke. The cigarette packages that announce higher risks of this or that age-related disease could cover all the risks by simply announcing that "Caution! Smoking Will Accelerate Aging and Increase the Probability of Your Early Mortality."

This warning, however accurate it may be, probably wouldn't stop anybody from smoking, of course—surprise! Nicotine is highly addictive, and most people can't stop even when they want to. Even the teenage girls or boys who start smoking at an early age and who then become aware they will get older faster (and probably get ugly faster) will still succumb to the peer pressures of the day, with the rationalization that "I can always stop in the future" (sadly, most of them can't).

While smokers will ignore the acceleration of the aging process, the acceleration of *mortality* is something that really is difficult to ignore. Just one example, osteoporosis, is worth thinking about since it is a condition that becomes rampant among smokers. Bones become thinner, much thinner, possibly contributed to by the smokers themselves being thinner (fatter people have stronger bones), or the smokers become more short-of-breath with exercise and therefore they are more sedentary (exercising people have stronger bones). Bones therefore break easier among smokers, as they also do more frequently in elderly people, who tend to have thinner bones and, unfortunately, who fall more frequently. Even if the acceleration of cancers, the *defining moment* for smokers, doesn't occur, hospitalizations for fractures alone are more frequent, and along with that, not surprisingly, mortality arrives sooner. By the age of about 40, it all starts to show—when I see a 40 year old person who looks 50—or more—it is virtually certain that person is a smoker, it is highly likely the bones are thin or are getting thin, that fractures will occur early leading to the hunched-over appearance of the elderly from thin crunched vertebrae.

Almost without exception, these people become shocked by the early arrival of their mortality.

Genetics always plays a role in the process of aging. As far as the acceleration of aging is concerned, we truly are what our genes dictate. And so, when there is a big difference in genes, as there is with different races, the effect on aging is profound. According to the Henry J. Kaiser Foundation,[10] Asians *living in the United States* live nearly eight years longer than Caucasians (86.5 vs. 78.9 years) and nearly twelve years longer than Blacks (86.5 vs. 74.6 years). Why do some races live so long and others live shorter lives? While variables in living circumstances (such as drug use or poverty differences between races) certainly plays a role, individual disease processes are also different between the races and have a profound effect on longevity.

For example, apparently because of specific genetic codes[11] that trigger prostate cancer, and a more aggressive form of the disease, Black men will be diagnosed with prostate cancer more frequently with an incidence of 255 compared to 161 in Caucasians, and they will die from the disease at a rate of 62 versus 25 for White males.[12]  Inadequate access to medical care in the early stages may also play role in this remarkable increased mortality.  Furthermore, Japanese women living in Japan have breast cancer only about ¼ as frequently as women in the United States (at the age of 60-64, there are 4900 breast cancer cases in Japan versus about 20,000 cases in the United States)[13]?  However, it must be said that while this might seem to be directly a race-related disease process, many other factors play a role in breast cancer, such as obesity, alcohol, and breast-feeding patterns.

But, as everything in biology, and as everything in medicine, the genetic role in the aging process is not so simple; the huge number of environmental variables at play continuously confounds the purity of genetics.  For example, regarding something we hear all the time, while the dismal statistic that life expectancy in the United States is about 40th in the world, compared to #1 Iceland and #2 Japan "in spite of the best care in the world" (a statistic and comment often used to promote socialized medicine), if you remove the crime-ridden areas of our inner cities or the high drug addiction factors in these cities, the data does not look nearly so bad for this country.  Furthermore, if you remove death by car accidents (and violent crime) from the international statistic tables of our country, longevity in the United States moves up to #1 in the world.[14]

Since all these variables play a role in determining when, exactly, each of us is likely to die, at what point in our lives should we start to think about throwing in the towel about survival?  At the age of 65 (or earlier) like the government wants us?  At 90, since that is by almost any measure *really* getting old?

Should age even be considered or should age be nothing more than just one of the myriad of factors that determines the best course of action when mortality is a possibility? Of course, age, as measured in years, is a consideration but *it should not be used as a primary factor behind deciding end-of-life issues.* We have seen how much variation there is among people all of the same age, and there is really no cut-off age beyond which it becomes appropriate to "pull the plug."

And so the conversation with Dr. Bosner in the emergency room continued.

"Everything else about Mrs. Pitsdale looks fine," he told me. "Regular rhythm, heart enzymes negative, blood pressure is normal, nothing cardiac that we can find. Anyway, she'll have to be admitted, okay for you to be the admitting doc?"

Of course all that was fine, since she *had* had a transient loss of consciousness, the cause had to be determined, and the potential reasons were innumerable. I placed her in the intensive care unit where everything including possible cardiac arrhythmias could be monitored. I completed her admission to the hospital and when I walked into her room, the nurse and her daughter, Scyrina, were helping Mrs. Pitsdale into a soft easy chair at the side of her bed.

The first words she said, as she rolled her eyes upward just as I came through the door were, "Whew! That always happens!"

"Now look, Mother," Scyrina said soothingly as she settled her mother into the chair, "Doctor Dunham is here and everything is going to be just fine!"

The tiny Filipino nurse looked up at me and said, "Ah, Doctor Dunham! We're just getting her out of bed for a bit."

"Roger! My boyfriend!" Mrs. Pitsdale exclaimed as she looked up at me, her wrinkled face beaming. "Are you here to save my life?"

"Evelyn, my sweetheart, I will save you," I said with a smile as her daughter patted her mother's arm and looked reassured. I gave the patient a stern look. "What is it that 'always happens,' like you were just saying, Evelyn?"

She looked puzzled for a moment and then her face lit up. "Oh, you mean just now, when I was getting into the chair?" She brushed her hand in a gesture of dismissal. "It's nothing, Roger, really nothing, just those Willies, they float through my head, and then they go away!"

Seeing that all was well, the nurse scooted out of the room as I glanced at the cardiac monitor above Mrs. Pitsdale. The wavy white line marching across the green monitor screen demonstrated a regular rhythm without any arrhythmias. I sat down with the two ladies, both of them a closely bonded family unit, and began to review her history and discuss the issue of blacking out. The patient lived alone at her own home in the back hills of Santa Barbara and Scyrina regularly provided her with transportation…to the stores for shopping, to my office, and once each year to the airport as they both departed for a week in France. The Willies had been with her about six months, she told me, each time lasting about ten or fifteen seconds, and almost always when she stood up from a chair or got out of bed. She had had a major Willie attack outside a store that morning, after standing, with the blackout immediately following and the daughter catching her before she hit the ground.

Ten minutes later, after the nurse and I completed the "postural blood pressure" measurements, we confirmed that her blood pressure dropped to a dangerous 65 or 70 with a major Willie-attack each time she stood. Furthermore, there were no increases in her heart rate, as should normally happen to keep her pressure up. It seemed that Mrs. Pitsdale was suffering from a severe postural hypotension syndrome, a condition that creates a high risk of blackouts with potential for falls and broken bones, a fairly common event in some diabetics, especially elderly ones.

I left the room, sat down in front of the computer at the nursing station, and began a mental debate as to what should be done next. I looked over her lab on the computer screen, all was normal. The sweet lady was 95 years old, what should I do? A cardiology evaluation? Added salt to her food, better hydration? A pacemaker, a treadmill, a heart scan? Special radioactive infusions to determine her coronary arteries' ability to carry blood to the muscle? A comprehensive chemical testing of her adrenal glands? Send her to a nursing home, with strict instructions to stay in bed all day? Almost everything sounded like a bad idea, although the pacemaker, with movement-sensing capability to speed up the heart when needed sounded feasible. I was certain the cardiologists would be happy to put one under the skin of her chest.

However, in the end, I gave her a pill, a tiny very cheap pill to be taken three times a day, a pill that can raise blood pressure, hopefully just the right amount, with some added salt and better fluid intake—just enough of that combination to keep her from the Willie-attack, but not so much to strain her heart. After a gentle treadmill check and a couple of days walking about the hospital with her nurse and daughter on each side, she joyfully declared herself to be freed from her dangerous friend Willie, she returned home and did perfectly well for another eight years, even returning to France a final time later that year.

At 103 years of age, a few months ago, her daughter couldn't get her into the car for an office visit one day, so I made a house call.

"Any more Willies?" I asked the frail woman lying in her bed.

"No, Roger," she answered weakly, her face crinkling into her sweet smile. "That Willie-guy hasn't come back…. I'm just getting weaker and weaker, it's getting too hard to get out of bed anymore." She smiled again and then looked serious. "Any ideas my dear boyfriend?" she asked.

A hundred things I could have done beyond the exam and routine blood tests drawn at home, things from nursing homes to physical therapy, things that would require the hospital, and things from an army of consultants. But when the blood tests and urine tests were essentially normal, and the conferences with her daughter and a more remote son were completed, it was clear that the best thing for this sweet 103-year-old lady was to keep her comfortable in her home, in her own bed, with a hospice nurse checking on occasion and her daughter checking regularly. Stopping the insulin, stopping any tests of blood sugars or anything beyond what would keep her comfortable, my elderly patient lived for two more weeks, able to say goodbye to her family, and then slowly slid down into a coma when the goodbyes were done, comfortable with her state of impending mortality, comfortable and contented right up to the final last breath and the final moment of her death.

Would that have been the right thing for her, or any other patient, at the age of 95?

For some, yes, but for others, no. When she was 95 years, Mrs. Pitsdale was too young. Was it right for a lady of 103? Yes, but only because she had, by that time, become too old. And not just because she was 103, but because anything else I might do would have just cost significant amounts of money, caused pain and suffering, and would never bring her back to her youth she was enjoying in her 90's and before.

# CHAPTER 4
## The Quality Dilemma:
## How Much Suffering is Too Much?

"I gotta gun, Doc, let me outta here," Larry Bradberry said to me, his burning eyes glaring across the room.

I looked at the pale 53-year-old man lying in the Catholic hospital bed, his anguished face filled with anxiety and pain, his voice angry as he struggled to resolve the news I had just given him. Bradberry had come to my office two days before as an urgent add-on patient in the afternoon. He had been squeezed into the schedule and he had doubled-over in the waiting room chair with abdominal pain. My medical assistant had brought him into our exam room and I gathered the details of his history. It started suddenly, he had told me, in the region just above his umbilicus, spreading around and gripping his mid-section like a hot vise that would not release. "I'm a smoker," he had reminded me, "I'm sure it's an ulcer or something like that. Smokers get ulcers, right? I'm sure it's not anything dangerous like lung cancer, not down here in my stomach. I took some antacids, didn't help, took Mylanta, got diarrhea, gets worse with food, and I can't eat."

I had finished his history and examined him, finding nothing more than a man with some weight loss and severe distress from a tender abdomen. I had outlined the anticipated hospital evaluation, starting with some blood tests, then further tests looking for intestinal blood loss, checking his white blood cell count, looking for anemia, gall bladder function, pancreas function, and some ultrasound studies. I had told him I was confident that, after we put him in the hospital, we would be able to find the answer within the next couple of days, and we could then plan an attack on whatever was creating his misery.

"Doc, you don't understand," Bradberry had blasted me, his forehead covered with sweat, his face grimacing from the pain. "I *know* pain, Doc, I've had pain before, lots of times. This is not *just pain*, this is a searing son-of-a-bitch bucket of lava, burning up my gut—I can't go on for 'a few days'—get me to the hospital ASAP, get me whatever drugs you have, find out what's wrong with me, and get a surgeon to cut this monster out of me!"

I had admitted him to the hospital within the next hour, high-speed to the medical floor, I had started him on some Fentanyl[15] while doing the tests, and when the ultrasound, followed by a CAT scan, showed something growing in the man's pancreas, I requested a surgeon do a quick biopsy—the frozen section confirmed pancreatic cancer.[16] At least, now, the intensity of his pain was explainable. The toxic digestive enzymes within the pancreas were dissolving his abdominal proteins in an intensely painful manner as the cancer caused them to leak out into the surrounding tissues. But his problem now, also explaining some of his 10-lb weight loss, was a primary malignancy that was spreading, disrupting his pancreas while sending long-reaching cancerous tentacles far out into the surrounding tissue like some kind of creature from hell. His chest x-ray had also revealed early spread of the cancer into his lungs, a spray of tiny metastatic nodules on both sides—he undoubtedly had many more tumors throughout the rest of his body, including his liver, his bones, and possibly his brain.

I had tried to reassure the man that everything possible would be done for him. An oncologist would see him and outline considerations for chemotherapy to slow the growth within the pancreas. The surgeon could not remove it, considering its far-reaching spread beyond the abdomen, not even with a heroic surgical procedure (called a "Whipple)[17]," but a cancer radiologist could provide a scientific outline of the radiation dose for him to further slow the growth. He would probably need to start on daily insulin, as his pancreas became more damaged from the tumor, creating a cancer-induced diabetes. Another radiologist would do a metastatic screening series with CAT scans clarifying lung and bone invasions, and a nuclear medicine physician would inject radioactive isotopes into his body, searching for further spread of microscopic tumor, beyond the visible tentacles. A nutritionist could guide him to a safer diet that would not stimulate his pancreas and that might add some pounds to his thinning body. We had somebody for everything, I told him, the best of scientific expertise to go on the attack.

"What about the pain, Doc?" he had asked, "and what are the chances of a cure?"

I hesitated, since I could not easily tell him what seemed to have become obvious. There was metastatic cancer growth beyond the pancreas, he was going to die from this cancer, I knew that, he almost certainly knew it, and he was probably going to die soon. I knew his future would include continuous unbearable pain including more of his severe episodes of "burning lava" excruciating pain. I knew that, with the proper orders, he would then begin receiving the armada of hospice care analgesics as he suffered and withered down the miserable path toward death, and I also knew that he would need ever-increasing doses of narcotics because he would quickly develop a buildup of drug tolerance.

The one very bad thing that stood out above it all: Larry Bradberry's mortality would involve an extraordinary amount of pain and suffering.

I hesitated again as he watched me intently. "We can help modify the pain, Larry..." I started before he interrupted me, his hollering voice again blasting me with the demand for his checkout to get his gun and end it all. And the words, "I have a gun," really have only one meaning in this setting—there was no doubt about what he was going to do with it, and likely use it promptly in his state of advance anguish. I could give him all the narcotics in the world, I could give him "medical marijuana" for whatever that was worth (now that it is legal in California), I could send him to an ancient cure-all clinic in India or Mexico, none would be helpful, all would just take his money without real benefit. His use of the gun would be a suicide, of course, and the words of medical school and hospital protocol and policy flashed through my mind — "If the subject exhibits a danger to himself or to others, intervention is lawfully justified…." is the way such well-meaning sentences started.

And so, what should I do? Check him out of the hospital so he can kill himself, ending the pain, ending the suffering? Was *that* the solution? Put him into an involuntary locked psychiatric ward with guards to protect him from himself? Call a palliative care consult? Or give him enough narcotics to do it himself, hoping his wife wouldn't call 911 after he moved into a prolonged coma and hoping his grown children wouldn't hold contempt for him for killing himself?

In medical school, some psychology-intervention professor might say something like, "It has become time for a psychiatrist, because the subject is getting depressed…."

Depressed? A psychiatrist? *Of course he's depressed, he's just been told he is going to die a miserable painful death from a rapidly spreading cancer!* This was not just a depressed man wanting to commit suicide, this was a man who was dying and who was searching for any escape from the misery of the process. All of it seemed pretty rational to me, and he was looking to his doctor for a solution.

I said nothing for about ten seconds after his repeated demand for release, I just looked at his anguished face and we both stared at each other in silence.

Finally, I asked softly, *"Have you thought about your wife?"* I waited a few seconds and then asked, "And, what about your children?"

My question hung in the air and then he suddenly covered his face with his hands and began sobbing. I went to the bedside and put my hand on his shoulder, and I gave him his answer.

"You're going to stay here, Larry, I'll take care of your pain."

He looked up at me as my words sank in. "You want me to stay here? You can take care of the pain for me?"

"There is almost no limit what I can do for you, here in the hospital," I said. "I will help resolve your pain with some of the best nurses on the planet and some of the best medicine ever invented for pain. You don't want a suicide to be the last memory about you in the minds of your wife and your children, you really don't want them to forever have the vision of what you did with your gun."

"But what about the surgeon? The radiology doc, the oncologist?"

"Nope. But one warning for you."

"What is that?"

"You will become constipated…." I smiled.

He wiped his eyes and looked at me again. "Constipation? That will become my biggest problem?"

"From the narcotics for pain control, but we have stuff for that." I paused and added, "You'll be here another week, or maybe a bit longer, I would guess."

His eyes widened slightly as the meaning of his time duration, *week or maybe a bit longer* for an end-of-life problem, sank in.

"Call your wife," I said, turning to leave. "Get her in here. Your time with her is more valuable than it has ever been. Also, there are no "visiting hours" here, she can stay as long as she'd like. Talk with her, spend time with her. And call your children—your wife will need their support."

"I didn't want my kids to know what..."

"Larry, your kids *need to know*," I said, "for their own sake as well as the sake of Mrs. Bradberry. Like I said, time is short."

For the next several hours, I ratcheted up his pain medication to provide him with nearly complete relief, moving him to levels well beyond the normal amount usually required for pain control, but not so much to prevent his clear thinking and conversation. Gratefully, there is no upper limit in setting the dose of narcotics in this kind of setting. There is a comprehensive set of policies that Medicare and insurance companies follow for the payment of care inside and outside the hospital at the end of life, but for Larry Bradberry (and many other patients), there were unique circumstances that required hospital attention. Also, if hospitalized Medicare patients enter the hospice program (requiring a determination of having less than 6 months left of life, no problem for Mr. Bradberry), there are dramatic changes regarding what is no longer "covered services," as follows:[18]

*"When you choose hospice care, you've decided that you no longer want care to cure your terminal illness and related conditions, and/or your doctor has determined that efforts to cure your illness aren't working. Medicare won't cover any of the following, once you choose hospice care:*

■ *Treatment intended to cure your terminal illness and/or related conditions. Talk with your doctor if you're thinking about getting treatment to cure your illness. You always have the right to stop hospice care at any time.*

■ *Prescription drugs (except for symptom control or pain relief).*

■ *Care from any provider that wasn't set up by the hospice medical team. You must get hospice care from the hospice provider you chose. All care that you get for your terminal illness and related conditions must be given by or arranged by the hospice team. You can't get the same type of hospice care from a different provider, unless you change your hospice provider. However, you can still see your regular doctor if you've chosen him or her to be the attending medical professional who helps supervise your hospice care.*

■ *Room and board. Medicare doesn't cover room and board. However, if the hospice team determines that you need short-term inpatient or respite care services that they arrange, Medicare will cover your stay in the facility. You may have to pay a small copayment for the respite stay.*

■ *Care in an emergency room, inpatient facility care, or ambulance transportation, unless it's either arranged by your hospice team or is unrelated to your terminal illness and related conditions. Note: Contact your hospice team before you get any of these services, or you might have to pay the entire cost."*

From this set of adrenaline-activating Medicare policies, if further care in the hospital could help this poor man (and I was quite certain that it could), then hospice care would do little more than deplete the life savings upon which his soon-to-be-widow would be needing. The hospital's Palliative Care Team would also seem to be of little value beyond what I already would be providing the patient--there was little to be gained from surrounding him with additional strangers, no matter how competent they might be. And so, a summary of my choices between these two end-of-life options below led to the conclusion that neither would work:[19]

| Hospital-Based Palliative Care Team | Hospice Agency Services |
|---|---|
| Patients can be at any stage of illness, from months to years | Patients have a prognosis of 6 months or less and a terminal diagnosis |
| Services provided in the hospital | Services provided in home, nursing home, assisted living, or hospice house |
| Reimbursed through existing channels | Reimbursed per diem under hospice benefit |
| Length of stay varies based on identified needs, therapies involved | Length of stay is 2 months on average; all therapies must have been completed |
| No bereavement services | 1 year of bereavement counseling |
| Does not use volunteers | Uses volunteers for family team members and bereavement support |

The primary considerations important in this case, from my perspective, were that the man's pain was severe and incapacitating, that his life expectancy was very short, that his wife was emotionally fragile and needed all the help she could get, that he had a primary care physician (me) who could spend time

53

with him and his family along the way with bereavement, counseling, and that further input *on top of the care he would already be receiving* was unnecessary.

I initiated a modified hospice-like plan, focused on pain relief, together with other orders to ensure no insurance company would even think about trying to kick him out of the Catholic hospital. I talked with the nurses, and left orders to ensure his nutrition was adequate and his bowel function would not cause distress. I wondered about the Catholic agenda of the hospital, and was quickly reassured by the Medical Staff Office that this treatment plan was well within religious guidelines to bring relief of pain even though the time of death may be sooner. It would be clear to all, including the kind Catholic Sisters in the hospital that it would be the malignancy that killed Mr. Bradberry, not the medicine that protected his evolving mortality from becoming a road to hell, as is the case with suicide. As I finished writing his orders, it was quite certain to me that the actual religious hell promised to Catholics and others who commit suicide would not apply here since I was giving him his morphine and his gun would remain safely locked up at home.

For the next week, Larry's wife spent hours at his bedside as the intravenous morphine allowed him to speak without the painful anguish from his tumor. They talked about everything on their minds, they discussed their marriage, their lives, and their love, they reviewed their finances, and they established a clear pathway for her future. A couple of children living far away, and now grown, appeared in his hospital room for further discussions, a priest offered religious salvations along the way, a Protestant minister stopped by to add some soothing words for the patient and his wife, while the nurses protected his skin with a soft air mattress and monitored the doses of medication.

He and I talked during my rounds in the hospital each morning, his thoughts offering me the kind of crystal-clear insights only a man who is dying can have. I assessed his pain regularly, and I increased his morphine as needed to protect him. And when he finally slid down into the inevitable coma as his kidneys shut down and the resultant uremia began to act like an anesthetic, he became comfortable within his dreams enclosed by the arms of Morpheus. At the end, Larry Bradberry found contentment in the evolution of his early mortality, and at the moment of his death, he was without suffering while surrounded by his family.

While I provided guidelines and a pathway for his mortality, the underlying diagnosis and the severe pain accompanying a spreading malignancy can ironically define a more certain pathway for a patient who finds him or her getting sucked down a vortex to the final event of death. The pain helps crystalize the decision-making process for the patient and the doctor regarding the critical question, what to do next? The pain removes many of the longer pathways (including in this case Palliative Care Team interventions and hospice), while sharpening the focus, both for the patient and for the patient's family, as well as for the doctor and the medical team. Without this certainty, without this focus, the process of improving mortality can go down many longer avenues, leading to delays, frustrations, interventions from many commercial entities, wasted money and suffering.

During my years of practice, while the inputs from patients have been as varied as the patients themselves, there are some general concepts that have emerged as a kind of medical truth about mortality. At the top of the list, heard over and over again from virtually every patient facing death is, *"I don't want to have pain, I don't want to suffer."* The gun for Bradberry was not because he wanted to kill himself. He had not been a depressed man, he had never even thought about suicide. He just wanted to end his terrible pain here and now if I couldn't do it…and he was a man of action. In his mind, if nobody else could help, then he would, by God, do it himself.

Often, however, the approaching mortality may generate pain that is more tolerable and then the other factors so common near the end of life become as important.

Additional elements that increase the burden of suffering also include, *"I want to maintain control of my circumstances,"* recognizing that the loss of control over what's happening, the loss of mental function adds great misery to the mortality process. It also means that that person, who may also be facing loss of ability to eat, to use the bathroom, to walk, and to interact with others in a coherent manner, wants desperately to not lose those quality elements of life so important. This factor alone rises clearly when any patient looks at the prospect of Alzheimer's disease or other neurological degenerative conditions associated with the loss of clear thinking ability.

Additionally, patients don't want to linger on a mortality pathway that goes on and on and on, indeterminately with very slowly increasing misery punctuated by the pain from a broken bone here or there, increasing breakdown of skin from pressure on mattresses, and the lonely consequence of relatives who no longer visit because of the unsettling debilities that accumulate. A long lingering progressively miserable pathway is also often associated with severely declining financial circumstances. Clearly, nobody wants to run out of money where, as reserves in bank accounts disappear, the quality of care inevitably declines.

Other factors from a long and lingering death are that self-respect vanishes if the care becomes limited because of diminished resources; the nurses who should be at the bedside can't be there because each has 20 patients instead of 5 or 6. Also, the inevitable result may often be that the patient gets dumped into a Medicaid-filled reservoir of immense human suffering, a mediocre nursing home environment filled with strong smells of fecal or urine containers that are unemptied, and a shortage of the kind of nurses who actually care about the collective nightmare of humanity that face them every day of their working lives.

Also, virtually nobody wants to die alone. It is almost an axiom of human existence that death is, almost by design, a frightening and lonely process. Standing on the edge of the cliff of life that drops away to the uncertain depths of the deadly unknown, an impending death is a uniquely individualistic event; two or more people may travel up to the edge, but only one person goes over the edge at a time. Death is *inherently lonely*. Furthermore, death should not be perceived more acceptable by the common random thoughts about others who might have died first, like *somebody I will be joining if I can find them*, irrespective of the logical challenge of trying to find other loved ones in a heaven holding billions and billions of people who have gone on before. Also, while there is a widespread belief that there is a sorting system *up* there; there is no such system perceived if the destination is *down* there.

Finding a departed loved one or friend in hell does not spark favorable thoughts

If there ever was a time to treasure the wife or the husband, the children or the grandchildren, the lover of decades or the others in life who have cared, the fact of an impending mortality gives an added powerful importance to these relationships. These are the people who will comfort you in your final weeks or days, who will oversee the caregivers who tend to the array of medical needs, who will speak softly into your ear when you might be slipping into a coma, barely able to hear or understand the powerful feelings that may surfacing. This is the time to treasure the relationship. If any human being, in a time of good health, has no such relationship, it would seem to be a good idea to get started building one....

If we should go out of this world like technology entrepreneur, visionary and inventor Steve Jobs did, it was a good thing for the loved one at his bedside to hear his final words[20], "Oh, wow! Oh, wow! Oh, wow!" and to respond with the most soothing final words he could ever hear during his remarkable lifetime.

The Living Will has, for several decades now, formalized and legally certified this process for easing the path to the end before that time arrives. This document, specific for each state in the country, is easily found on the Internet and the wording addresses this need:

*I do not want my life to be prolonged if (1) I have an incurable and irreversible condition that will result in my death within a relatively short time, (2) I become unconscious and, to a reasonable degree of medical certainty, I will not regain consciousness, or (3) the likely risks and burdens of treatment would outweigh the expected benefits,*

The term "condition" is essential to this process, requiring that there be a medical certainty; also, this condition must in fact be "irreversible" and this condition "will result in my death." These elements are also needed when anybody considering suicide is trying to plan a decent mortality process in the face of overwhelming disease, and this is where the laws in different states allowing such suicide, the so-called "right-to-die" laws, need to be examined carefully.

The Living Will is a legal document, requiring witnesses or notary certification, for it gives direction on a matter that, when it is over, is obviously irreversible. When another patient of mine, an elderly man we'll call Mr. George Stanwood, became increasingly short of breath one night because of his underlying emphysema, the nurses called me around midnight, telling me the family was concerned about his distress and inquiring whether he should be on a respirator. With his long history of high carbon dioxide levels and low oxygen levels, it was clear that he would never be able to come off the respirator if he was ever put on one.  Also, because he had filled out the Living Will, it was clear that he did not want his life prolonged by such mechanical interventions and that the "burdens of treatment would outweigh the expected benefit."  The additional problem was that he would have to be transferred to the intensive care unit, (where visiting hours are limited) and that he already had had virtually every medicine for emphysema brought to him by superbly competent pulmonary physicians. There was really nothing more that could be done.  The nurses wanted to know where it was *in writing* that these directions against mechanical intervention existed—otherwise, they said, he would "have to immediately be transferred to the intensive care unit for intubation and respirator support."

My high-speed drive to my office late that night to fax Mr. Stanwood's Living Will to the nursing station allowed him to receive narcotic medicines in a quiet room on the general medicine hospital wing that lessened his distress and allowed his impending mortality to lead to a peaceful one several days later.[21]

These doctor-assisted suicide desires can be fraught with uncertainty.  Take for example the 23-year-old woman who comes into a doctor's office and announces that "Doctor, because of..." (fill in the blank) I have determined that I am suffering too much and the time has come for me to go.  I want one of those suicide pills that you can now legally give me!"  Any licensed doctor with decent credentials will want to know the diagnosis actually extends beyond depression, or possibly psychosis, and that self-inflicted death or doctor-assisted death is not just inappropriate and illegal suicide or just plain murder. This would seem that this kind of thing could be easily managed but in fact it is not so easy and, fortunately, the laws in the various states allowing patient suicide actually do have conditions to prevent exactly this kind of depression-related event.

Little of this information is handed to doctors-in-training, to be absorbed and implemented the day the MD degree is granted. There are too many variables for even the most robust training program to teach student doctors the proper pathway in every case. There is, therefore, not a streamlined pathway to the end...challenges to the concept of a single format, a single defined road, for a decent mortality are everywhere!

As an unusual mortality pathway, take my patient Mr. Jackson, for example. His wife, a lovely lady who had been an excellent wife for nearly forty-five years came home one evening and found this note on their front door from her husband:

*"I am out back, but you won't like what you're going to find."*

And so, with considerable trepidation, she went around the house to the back yard and found her husband lying back on a lounge chair after having just shot himself in his head. Like many patients who try such terrible things, he had shot himself in a manner that he thought would be associated with instant death, but he found instead that he was just suddenly transformed into a man who suddenly became severely brain damaged. If he had problems before, his problems now were considerably worse.... With the gun on the tile decking next to him, Mr. Jackson was still alive but bleeding from his head wound, and neurologically a disaster with brain damage and the inability to talk or to function much beyond labored breathing.

Mrs. Jackson almost fainted away at the sight, but she had enough composure to call the paramedics and then my cell phone. I came to the emergency room where the ER doctor and I shook our heads in a gesture of collective medical dismay. I admitted him to a quiet corner of the hospital with a protocol to ensure he did not continue this life for more than a day, or maybe two at the most. I spent much more time consoling and calming Mrs. Jackson and her daughter than I spent with the patient. I reviewed the CT (computerized tomography) X-ray scans with a very unhappy neurosurgical consult to confirm the man was *irreversibly* brain-damaged and would die in a short period of time with or without the morphine I started pumping into his veins. The next day, in that quiet corner of the hospital, Mr. Jackson died from his self-inflicted wound…I just helped him along the way, but it was a miserable mortality for Jackson and his entire family.

He had been a man depressed, he had steadfastly refused psychiatry consult requests for more than two years, he had refused to take his anti-depressant medicine, and in the end, he suffered greatly, he made his wife and daughter suffer greatly, and his mortality was an abysmal disaster process. The cause of it all? Endogenous depression, usually significantly treatable if treatment would be allowed. It was not in this case, and the end result was a tragedy not only to the patient, but by his own doing, a tragedy that left for all of his family an eternity of unspeakable memories.

Then there was Mr. Swanson with his colon cancer, cared for during my training years by an oncologist, Dr. Blackstone. The man had been declining overall with worsening symptoms, but still had some reasonable quality of life remaining. He had developed a relatively mild blood infection, he had been put in the hospital and I examined him as a "physician in training," working as a medical resident. I wrote the orders for his limited diet, for his intravenous antibiotics, and for a couple of tests I wanted performed the next morning. The tests were never done since Dr. Blackstone ordered the nurses to give the man something he later told me was a "goodbye suppository." The pharmacy mixed up the meds, the nurse inserted the suppository into the patient's rectum, and ten minutes later, Mr. Swanson was dead. As the 30+ years have since gone by since that day, I could never get out of my mind how a physician could make a decision (perhaps privately discussed with the patient, I'll never know) that right now, here today, the time has come to change a relatively peaceful mortality process into a remarkably instant death. The rationale perhaps was that the man was going to die anyway, and now look at all the pain and suffering he wouldn't go through.

This seemingly arbitrary and capricious act *by a physician* underscores the potential risks to patients empowered with the same ability to do this to themselves under the "right to die" considerations of evolving common law. It is obvious that anybody suffering and in pain will have some bad days that, with the additional distress from an approaching mortality process, there could be an intensification of suicidal thoughts—perhaps on a day after a spouse became argumentative, perhaps after a bad night's sleep, or perhaps during a rainstorm where gloom and doom seemed to be everywhere. And although the common legal mandate of a double-oversight process (two physicians signing off the giving of lethal drugs to a patient) would seem to lessen the abuse of such a process, there seems little defense for doing something that might be arbitrary and yet is fundamentally irreversible.

As a not-too-hard-to-imagine possibility, what about the patient who then, on a down day, gives himself or herself a goodbye suppository *and then suddenly has a change of heart*? This brings to light a study done many years ago that asked the 26 or so survivors[22] who tried to leap to their deaths off the Golden Gate Bridge, *and had survived*, what percent of them had a "change of heart on the way down?" Since more than 1600 bodies have been recovered from jumping from this bridge (the second-leading structure-associated suicide structure in the world, just below the Nanjing Yangtze River Bridge in China, and determined to be 98% fatal), it is interesting that of those who actually survived the impact, nearly all of them regretted having taken the big leap. One of the survivors, Kevin Hines, was quoted as saying, "There was a millisecond of free fall. In that instant, I thought, what have I just done? I don't want to die. God, please save me." Furthermore, most of the 118 potential jumpers who were talked out of leaping in the first place never went on to commit suicide. This gives one pause when the "patient-assisted suicide" issues are discussed—the fall from the bridge to impact with the water takes about 4 seconds, the time after the insertion of such a suppository is generally more than 5 minutes....

The Oregon experience with doctors' prescriptions for patients wanting to end their lives is instructive. In the past 17 years, doctors in that state have written 1,173 prescriptions[23] for patients who decided the time was right for them to end their lives. However, with the prescriptions in hand, more than 400 of these patients *did not* use the lethal drugs...a new day, the sun came out, a change in heart, a decision to "continue on," the reasons are not known and have not been adequately studied. Also, of the 752 patients who did use the medication and definitely died from the medication, there is no record of how many changed their minds after taking the drug overdose. If a patient did change his or her mind and decided not to die, and yet the doctor had ensured the patient would definitely die, shouldn't there be some responsibility on the medical profession to examine the ethics of terminating a patient's life, a patient who might decide, belatedly perhaps, that an accelerated death was not a good idea? And, really, what could be worse than a patient deciding to take a lethal dose of his or her prescribed goodbye medication, who then decides that was a bad idea, who then desperately tries to reverse the effect but then dies anyway?

As of this writing, California now has an assisted-suicide law (passed during a special session by the legislature seeking to "find funding" for healthcare programs). California voters had rejected this lethal drug prescribing law in 1992, 2005, 2006, and 2007; the "special session" effectively bypassed the voters, and the law then went into effect in 2016. The assisted-suicide termination of life is also allowed in Washington, Vermont and Montana, although in Montana it was by a court decision. The data in California is now being gathered.

The simple question, then, has never been answered in any state: if a physician is allowed to kill a patient with a prescription drug, shouldn't there be a fail-safe backup plan (for example, a narcotic antagonist) for those patients who change their mind after taking the drug? The Oregon experience suggests there might be as many as a third of the patients, those who had previously requested a lethal drug (during a moment of desperation) and then never took the drug. How many were there, exactly, who took the drug and *then* changed his or her mind?

Also, if a physician is allowed to easily kill his or her patient, what about an extension of this process to a relative who might gain an earlier inheritance, a policeman with a dislike of this or that person, or a neighbor with a long-smoldering grudge—when does this taking of life ever become murder? There seems to be no practical limit to the consequences of a state-sponsored green light for the termination of life, primarily because of the demonstrated uncertainty patients may have about such a profound and irreversible event. Also, has anybody ever documented the "dignity" aspect of the lethal drug—do these people taking the drug really die with an aura of dignity or do they go through the suffering that I have seen so many times and that hospice nurses treat regularly in their dying patients?  Only one thing is certain—patients whose lives are ended early save the state millions of healthcare dollars, and considering today's widespread budget shortfalls, does this not (at least subconsciously, perhaps) enter into the minds of legislators or governors as they ponder or promote such laws?

With all this in mind, is it not surprising how easy it is for a patient to fill out a single one-page form to end his or her life?  For example, in the state of Washington and Oregon, the forms are virtually identical—a single page with a fill-in-the-blanks set of questions.  The patient attests that he or she is "of sound mind" (no documentation needed), that a specific terminal condition is present, confirmed by a "consulting physician" (with "terminal event" credentials…the pathologist Jack Kevorkian comes to mind) and that the expected "results" are "known" (the word "death" is noted later). The opportunity to inform (or to not inform) family members is initialed, the elements of "moral responsibility" are accepted for the action (meaning the morality to kill oneself is nobody but the patient's responsibility), and finally it is noted that the awaited death "may take longer" than anticipated…. Although it is observed that the patient has the "right" to rescind the request and to decide NOT kill oneself, there is no mention of what happens if the impending death is without "dignity," or if the impending death does not occur at all (should one take *more* lethal drugs, maybe try again later)?  There is no mention about what should be done if the patient *changes his or her mind after the drugs are taken*.  If the "expected death" doesn't occur in three hours, or if the patient decides a few more goodbyes would be a good idea *after the drug is taken,* what then?  When prisoners on death row fail to be executed in spite of extensive efforts by the executioners, and when distressed patients jumping from the Golden Gate Bridge change their minds in 4 seconds after the leap, did anybody who crafted this process in these states think about the moral and practical debacle inherent with this process? And are the physicians who are a party to this collusion of this attempted self-execution "with dignity" not aware of their own ability to do their job and work with hospice and other excellent nursing systems who support a genuine dignity in the final days or moments?

These considerations alone suggest the lurking of a most unsavory spectrum inherent within the patient-assisted suicide laws. Perhaps some leadership is needed in the states of Vermont, Montana, Washington, Oregon, and California for the people to understand the downside of self-execution and for the doctors to expand awareness of their ability to ease the pain and suffering at the end of the mortality pathway.

# CHAPTER 5
## How Do You Plan for the *Unknown*?

It is easy to plan for the certainty of death, but the uncertainty of mortality is another story. A perfect example of the challenge was the jolting case of Missy Cartel. Slumped down in her wheelchair, she was pushed by her attendant through the front door of my office one afternoon, a thin, pale, wealthy and reluctant 52-year-old woman, delivered from Los Angeles as directed by her attorney. The patient was frightened as the attendant guided her 97 curled-up pounds to my back office for the gathering of her medical history and the preparation for an examination. She clutched the arms of the wheelchair with tiny thin hands, she had jet-black hair with a mixture of premature gray and her sad blue eyes were sunken back into a face that showed evidence of substantial weight loss.

As her wheelchair aligned across from my office chair, I instructed the attendant to depart the room and wait for us in the front office. This was going to be a strictly private affair, private to all, that is, but her Los Angeles attorney, a Mr. Mike Sill, her only trusted confidant in the world, a lawyer friend from my own childhood who was active in providing clients with legal advice regarding wills, trusts, and benefits.

"Welcome to my office," I said to her pleasantly and asked if she would like some water.

"No, I don't want any water and I don't want to be here," she promptly answered, her voice abnormal, high-pitched, and spoken with difficulty. "Mike forced me to come. He said I need a diagnosis or my trust payments won't be given to me. I really don't want to be here," she repeated. "I only trust Mike."

"Okay, I understand, I'll try to make this easy for you," I told her. "Maybe we can get the correct diagnosis and make your problems improve…."

"I don't think so," she answered softly. "Furthermore, I don't *want* to know what's wrong with me and I don't *want* to be here."

"I understand. Have any other doctors seen you?"

"No," she snapped as she closed her eyes for a moment, like she was trying to shut me out of her mind.

My mind raced ahead—her speech was not normal, that was obvious. It had a strange and subtle scanning quality with a disrupted flow of words and longer than normal pauses between syllables. Also, there was a slight slurring of her words. From the thinning of her muscles in her arms and legs (provoking the need for the wheelchair), it was clear a medical disaster had long been underway. The weight loss (of about 50 pounds) had been worsening over the past year or so, but her problem speaking had been a continuing problem for at least the past two years.

With considerable difficulty and gentle guidance, I was finally able to obtain the complete story of her decline. She lived alone near Beverly Hills, and she had preferred to be alone most of her life. Missy was a classic "loner," she just didn't enjoy being around people. She was extremely wealthy as the sole beneficiary of some trust that her attorney was monitoring and apparently money had never been a problem. When she gradually became so debilitated that she couldn't answer the telephone in her luxury suite, Mr. Sill visited her and mandated a live-in caregiver plus some strict instructions to be driven north and to appear in my office for an examination.

"Mike told me I need a diagnosis," she told again me in her strange speech pattern. "He will pay you whatever your fee is, now let's get this over with," she concluded as I prepared for the examination.

With the help of my two medical assistants, we managed to get her up on the exam table, I documented a vast array of neurological problems, we wheeled her across the street to the hospital for a MRI scan, and the diagnostic pattern of MS (multiple sclerosis) was confirmed. Her brain was filled with plaques from this insidious disease, and clinically, the damage was profound, likely to be irreversible. After her return to Los Angeles that afternoon, I called her with the news and the recommendations that the Neurological Department at UCLA see her to perform a spinal tap for the clarification of the activity of her immune system, helping confirm the diagnosis and to prepare for treatment. She absorbed the news with near-silence, she refused to go to UCLA, she refused the spinal tap, and she made it clear that she did not want to know anything more. I tried to encourage her and she started crying.

"Why can't you understand?" she finally said, somewhat breathlessly. "I don't *want* to know anything more!"

She then broke off contact with me, preferring to struggle on with the help of her assistant and the continuing infusions of money controlled by Mr. Sill.

Clearly, Missy Cartel simply did not want to know. When she had first lost her vision for two days a couple of years before, only to have it return again, she had freaked out but even then, she did not want to know why; her vision returned to nearly-normal and she felt reassured that everything would be okay. When her speech gradually began to change, she found she could still communicate satisfactorily and she still did not want any answers. The weakness of her muscles, the weight loss, all created the same response. She could get along, so leave me alone was the general thinking pattern. All along this path, she knew the answers would alarmingly define her mortality, and clearly it would be an accelerated mortality from something awful that was going on in her brain. Missy absolutely did not want to know because she did not want to directly look at the harsh reality of her mortality. Like a stick floating down a river that begins to accelerate as it approaches something creating a loud roaring noise, she wanted to ignore it all, and to allow herself to just float along, right up to the falls and beyond.

*Besides, the water really wasn't moving all that fast at this time, at least it didn't seem to be....*

The worst thing about not wanting to know was that there could be no planning in this crumbling world of Missy Cartel. She could not plan because she did not *want* to know what was going on in her body and what terrors it represented about her future. At her young age, the alarming symptoms should have been a call for her to gather information about what was in her future, a future with a shortened lifespan she strongly suspected, but at the same time, a future that would create problems beyond her ability to accept. To plan any element of mortality required that she understood what was coming—what was eventually coming, however, was decline and death, so frightening that she simply blocked it out of her mind. Without her attorney, she would have been perfectly happy to just continue on to the very end, doing what she could as she progressively could do less. She had struggled on, finally and inevitably needing the help of the assistant, but all the way down this pathway of horrors, she could not plan because she had managed to entirely screen out the concept of knowing her own mortality.

To most young and healthy people, the whole concept of mortality is an abstraction…sure, there are lots of things that can get me, he or she may think, but right now I feel great, I'll stay away from high-speed motorcycles, and I don't want to worry about it. For many people, around the age of fifty or so, when memory starts to fade a little or become less reliable, the chilling consideration of Alzheimer's disease begins to enter the mind with all its unacceptable consequences relating to a difficult and an uncertain planning process. Then, as time continues to pass, if any strange or new symptoms develop, there is an inclination to start seriously considering, and gradually accepting, the concept of mortality—a practical result especially since *immortality* is not readily feasible (or, to most, even desirable), and since, if an earlier death is to be avoided, there needs to be additional thinking and planning.

Again, planning for death is relatively easy. My parent's plan for their deaths was specific and exact. They defined and printed out the directions with instructions for their children that, when each of them died, the Neptune Society would take their bodies, turn them to ashes, and cast the ashes into the waters of the Pacific Ocean. That was what was done in each case. We called the Neptune Society operator, a mortician arrived, and about two weeks later, a death certificate showed up in the mailbox with a letter confirming that everything was done as directed. My parents and the ocean had been joined as they had directed and Neptune had made it easy.

Simple.

But *what leads up to death*, the mortality process, is vastly more complicated because there are so many variables, there is so much emotion, and there can be so much potential for suffering. One size, such as cremation or a burial plot, does not fit all, and any one definition of, or guidance into, the mortality process will be wrong more often than right. Ten sizes will fit, maybe, two or three people, and thousands of sizes are available that may fit a few more. We have seen poor Mr. Joseph Tomascas hollering "Don't let me die!" as his aorta bled and his heart stopped in the elevator—no time for him to plan anything except to call 911 and to then hope for the best...as the worst rapidly

74

materialized and his unplanned mortality rapidly descended upon him. On the other side of the spectrum, I have seen so many people who have had more than a decade to plan, contrasting sharply with those like Mr. Tomascas. There is the Golden Gate Bridge with its 4-second pathway to oblivion and the man with the Goodbye Suppository with ten, fifteen, maybe twenty minutes to think about it and maybe change his mind. The variables apply to each and every one of these people.

And, there are the patients in Washington, Vermont, Montana, Oregon, and now California, gathering to take their "Death with Dignity" drugs, giving each of them just enough time to mull the approaching *irreversible* fate as the Great Reaper accelerates his Train of Death down the tracks and prepares for another unscheduled stop.

Yet, in today's world of advanced diagnostic tools, there is often plenty of time to plan the approach of mortality—and the planning is essential to improving the quality of life ahead. Isn't the compelling need to plan the very essence of the human spirit? Beyond the planning for the next meal, a fundamental characteristic seen across the entire animal kingdom, humans instinctively go beyond…far beyond…to plan all the elements we see as essential to each given day. We wake up in the morning and we have a plan in place—we have a *schedule* beyond breakfast, beyond the morning newspaper, beyond the regular bathroom break. We plan and we plan and we plan, at work, at play, with the gathering of money or the spending of money, all of it planned, all of it organized. This planning is based on assumptions largely governed by experience or lessons we have learned from our individual pasts and from those with experience. With big plans, *life plans,* we know for example that if we want to obtain a decent standard of living, it will be necessary to attend some kind of a training program, from trade schools to college and beyond to learn the necessary skills for a financially productive life. In the meantime, each of the small plans we make each day, the thousands of them, are designed to create a better life for ourselves or for those we love.

But, what about planning for mortality?

Few of us really have any experience with mortality; we've not done it before, there are few lessons available during our lives and yet planning for it is critically important. When should we start planning? Clearly the structured universe in which we all dwell can suddenly become fragmented when the prospect of mortality arises, where a point is abruptly defined beyond which the future ends, the point beyond where there can be no further plans because there is no life. The shock of this filled Missy's eyes as she struggled to speak of her neurological disassembly during the progression of her disease—she hadn't planned on any of that and the reality was more than she could comprehend. For those who seek answers to explain symptoms, the moment often arrives in a doctor's office, when the physician alarmingly hesitates, perhaps clears his throat, before revealing the results of a CAT scan, of a biopsy, or a diagnostic blood test—that frightening hesitation that can drive the patient to suddenly break out in a sweat and begin grappling with a new, and often terrifying, reality.

Even more terrifying, especially for those without a good physician, is the recognition of an accelerated mortality that is self-discovered on the Internet, as symptoms are Googled and studied with underlying fear. Furthermore, we are all cursed with a strange, nearly *automatic*, assumption as those of us with new symptoms read about various conditions that might or might not represent our "new disease," that the worst possible condition is precisely the one barging into a previously happy life. The usual lifeline of previous experience is of no value since the approach of mortality generally only happens once in a lifetime.

To make matters worse, the brighter we are and the more education we have, the worse this auto-selection-of-the-worst-diagnosis becomes. Take medical students for example, or take me when I was a medical student, as an example. My skin began to twitch one day, I noticed during a long lecture at the UCLA School of Medicine. The twitch on the arm was to be ignored, and then a twitch started on the side of my face, ignored again as I waited for it to disappear. And then twitching of the muscles on a leg, and again on my other arm, on and on. The more I thought about it, the more I twitched! Finally, that evening, with exasperation and the recognition that I was going to be a doctor and that I therefore could gather any information about anything I wanted, I researched the cause of twitching. In less than one minute of study, I came across the disease ALS (Lou Gehrig's disease), as we saw in poor Dr. Peter Jackson as he gazed his final gaze at the lights in the harbor below. The book made it clear, frighteningly clear, that "the disease can start insidiously with the twitching of the skin." As I broke out in a sweat, the twitching *increased*, as if my hypochondriacal body wanted to agree with my self-diagnosis.  The next day I scheduled an urgent visit with a competent UCLA neurologist to see if anything could be done to allow life to continue in spite of the inevitable decline.  He listened to my story, he thumped my reflexes, he tested my sensation ability and my muscle strength and then he sat back in his chair to drop the final diagnosis on me, the words that would forever define my mortality.

"Dunham," he said seriously and *without hesitation*, "back off on the coffee."

I walked out of the room feeling like I had just escaped the electric chair, my future was bright again, I *actually would* finish medical school in another couple of years and I *actually would* become a doctor.  The planning for my mortality could be delayed for a few more years, and best of all, the twitching seemed to fade away….

· So, the question must be asked:  is it really possible for anybody to ever plan for mortality?

It won't help to review the 4-inch thick textbook of pathology, or (for the millennial generation) the gigabytes of computer data organizing the variance of human disease.  A perusal of these pages quickly makes it clear how nearly impossible it is to plan the future before the problems leading to that mortality begin to surface.  On top of that, it's a bit ghoulish to even try…just living the adventure of life is really a lot more fun.  Furthermore, this is not exactly dinner table conversation, these are not thoughts to be casually shared with the family.  Missy Cartel was the perfect example of someone suspecting an emerging horror from within and not wanting to move to any kind of plan—still in her fifties, still too young to even *think* about such things.

Beyond the challenges of planning something so variable, from the physician's standpoint, when all is said and done, it is critical there also should be no regrets among the living when it is over. That means there has to be certainty that death, in fact, *really* is coming in spite of the best medical efforts to prevent it, and that it will come because of a defined and relentless disease that cannot be reversed. An actual disease mechanism must be defined, if for no other reason than to have a good idea how much time is available. This also requires the exclusion of hypochondriasis, where (in the mind) death lurks around every corner, mortality is coming fast and the future is a disaster. If it is determined that mortality really is approaching, is it time to review the writings of Dr. Elisabeth Kübler-Ross[24] in an effort to give structure to the planning process? If the mortality process really comes in stages, as she says, is it a good idea to memorize them so we're ready as they arrive?

The answer, in a word, is no.

Looking at the five stages defined by Dr. Kübler-Ross, we find the acronym DABDA, representing Denial, Anger, Bargaining, Depression, and Acceptance. Through interviews with patients facing death, this psychiatry physician summarized the experiences and categorized them in a compelling manner that opened the door for discussion about something that had previously been widely suppressed. For that reason alone, she deserves high accolades. Her work turned the spectrum of emotions being endured by dying patients into concise "stages," as she made an effort to create patterns of social science to explain the gamut of feelings previously seeming to be a complete morass of emotional debris.

It has been my experience, while caring for patients looking at their evolving mortality and their approaching death, that her definition of categories or "stages," as well as the implication that these arrive one after another (one develops as the previous one disappears?) are in conflict with almost all elements of medical reality. Furthermore, her stages not only do not necessarily arrive in any order, they may not arrive at all depending on the intelligence and emotional stability of the suffering individual, and greatly depending on the support mechanisms available such as family or capable counselors. The stages may equally apply to other life crises such as for children grieving the divorce of their parents, the loss of a loving relationship, or a myriad of issues relating to substance abuse. The stages may never arrive if mortality moves rapidly, or if the disease process can be modified, fought, or challenged to the greatest possible extent. Also, her credibility has come into question because of her bizarre departure into a pattern of delving into ideas relating to the hereafter in the 1970's, such as what happens after death including communications with the dead and "out-of-body" experiences, after-life, spiritualism, and mediumship[25]

Finally, her work seems to equate mortality with death, a conjoining of these entities which denies the distinctions previously defined in this book; also, the perception of mortality can exist in some individuals throughout much of their lives, or just in their senior years, without death arriving at all…or at least not for a long time. Probably the best characterization of Dr. Kübler-Ross' book written by one of the many readers who was described in the forward of the 40th Anniversary Edition of *On Death and Dying*, by Dr. Allan Kellehear[26]: "*On Death and Dying* has regularly been mistakenly and mischievously construed as a research study. It is a popular book of description, observation, and reflection based on a series of dialogues with dying people."

If there are not stages arriving in well-defined packages, and we cannot expect any or all stages to arrive as we age and the arrival of mortality becomes increasingly evident, what can be planned and what seems to work the best to help survival during the mortality process in times of challenge? Planning anything requires a clear mind; unfortunately, it is a reality that the planning process is profoundly affected by whether or not dementia is a part of mortality. We live inside our minds, all of us, and when a disorder evolves that deteriorates and destroys our ability to think, and a whole different array of planning is required.

Before it happens, however, how do we know if we're going to get dementia? How do we know whether this vital part of our "self" will move into a state of havoc, confusion, and disarray? There are some predictive indicators, such as strong family histories of Alzheimer's disease, a personal history of repetitive head trauma, a very long life all the way to becoming extremely aged, or a substantial history of drug abuse (including alcoholism); however, any or all of these indicators may be present and dementia never occurs.  If it does develop, dementia is a terrible circumstance of life since any further planning concepts fall to others.   And, what do I regularly hear from the distressed relatives of a demented person, a person who has reached a vegetative state, somebody needing regular diaper changes, a person requiring feedings from a caregiver, perhaps while staring blankly for hours at daytime television programs or staring at nothing at all?

"Good God!!!" these relatives say to me, sometimes as a group, "I *know* he never wanted to go on living like this, doctor, isn't there *something* we can do?"

*Isn't there something we can do?*

Actually, there are several things that cannot be done, since murder is not only illegal but also fundamentally *wrong*.  Of even greater importance is the acknowledgement that patients are not always like this, vegetating and waiting for a diaper change, they *become* like this over a period of time—a long time if the disease is Alzheimer's, but sometimes over a short time if you consider the cases of my unfortunate patients, Margaret Bottingham and Teresa Adams.

Mad Cow Margaret and Tattoo Teresa both had well-functioning minds, right up until the time abruptly arrived when they didn't.  Margaret Bottingham had been a very proper English lady of 63 years who began having challenges remembering certain fundamentals, such as her husband's name, where she kept her clothes, or where she lived.

"She forgot where I was yesterday," a distressed George Bottingham told me one day, as I interviewed them and prepared to examine her. "I was at work," he added, "at my office, where I've gone for the past twenty-three years!"

I glanced at Margaret's mini-mental status[27] test I had given her six months before, the routine test of mental function I give all my patients annually above the age of 60; it was perfectly normal. I looked at her thyroid screening studies and her other blood studies from three months before, all normal.

"Anything else going on?" I asked her husband as Margaret, sitting next to him, smiled and looked perfectly content.

"Well, yes..." he hesitated and then finally blurted out. "She gets really moody now, she no longer wants to be affectionate with me, and..."

"Oh, George!" Margaret promptly interrupted with an embarrassed laugh, playfully backhanding her husband's shoulder. "That's silly!" she added.

"She doesn't call our kids any more. She had always called them every week."

"I just forget, sometimes," she said more seriously, her dark eyes studying my face. "I'm perfectly fine, doctor, really, George just gets worried because I'm getting older."

I asked a few more questions and mulled over the possibilities, including pseudo-dementia,[28] a hematoma (blood clot of some kind) in the skull or brain, and an array of other dementia-causing conditions. I gave her another mini-mental status test, which she flunked, and a complete neurological exam, which was, otherwise, normal. When I finished with everything, it was clear that she had a serious problem with her thinking, a problem like Alzheimer's disease, but considering how rapidly the change was occurring, it almost seemed like Alzheimer's disease on a fast track. Margaret Bottingham was otherwise perfectly normal in every way I could detect. I decided to request an MRI scan of her brain, which was equivocal, and some more blood studies to look for any metabolic disorders. These follow-up studies were all normal, but as I called Margaret and her husband to tell them the good news, I noted that she had had all of her vaccinations brought up to date nine months before, and that I had prepared a Travel Sheet for her biennial trip to Great Britain.

Margaret Bottingham *regularly* traveled to Great Britain.

During that decade, Great Britain had been feeding their cows protein-containing foods from neurological remnants of diseased cows, mixed with their usual alfalfa, and the cows were increasingly becoming demented.[29] Also, and sadly for this very nice lady during one of her trips, she had consumed some beef that turned out to be infected (cooking the meat does not eliminate the infective agent). Two weeks later, UCLA confirmed from her spinal tap the presence of the characteristic abnormal proteins in her spinal fluid, the proteins indicating the presence of so-called prions[30] of Creutzfeldt-Jakob disease (CJD) or more commonly known as "Mad Cow Disease." This so-called CJD is a disaster to the mind, and created a situation where a healthy individual like Margaret Bottingham, without any known predisposing predictor of dementia, could rapidly become demented. Furthermore, there is no treatment for this disease, and she was, sadly, dead within a year.

Teresa Adams was another very nice lady of 56 years, also with some very bad luck. She and her husband regularly travelled to a desert city in Southern California to enjoy the balmy weather, the relaxed lifestyle, and various spa treatments. After one of her massages, she decided to visit an upscale tattoo parlor to allow for a subtle cosmetic tattooing of darkening ink across her eyebrows. When she returned to her home and presented a week or so later in my office for a physical exam, I noticed her eyebrows looked great but her skin had a classic waxy-yellow appearance suggesting the jaundice of hepatitis. Her blood studies confirmed she was suffering from Hepatitis C, and at that time, the much more advanced drug Solvaldi[31] was not available. The public health system in California raided the tattoo parlor but found no evidence of any Hepatitis C source, nor any proof of shoddy sterility practices; the actual source of her infection was never confirmed. Teresa ended up undergoing a treatment program for the Hepatitis C with Interferon, a drug that shows significant benefit stopping the replication of the virus but which has also been associated with the development of dementia. Her hepatitis improved, her viral counts dropped to a satisfactory level, but she abruptly began to become progressively demented.

Dementia at any age is terrible, but at 56? Especially when it arrives for in a relatively young person, when it progresses rapidly, and even worse when it might have been caused by *treatment* for a disease (although Hepatitis C in older patients is, itself, associated with the development of dementia). We could treat her hepatitis but there was no cure for the dementia; the only treatment was supportive. I had the unfortunate responsibility, along with her husband, of guiding her into nursing homes as she moved into a worsening condition and finally suffered a rapid demise from the complications of dementia.

Without dementia, planning is easier, primarily because of the cooperative interactions the patient may provide with those who care (both medical and family). My patient, Miguel Hernandez, was an example of this. With his failing heart from a narrowed aortic valve, this 83-year-old man with a loving wife and grown children struggled to stay alive. His congestive heart failure slowly progressed, however, he passed through some *but not all* of Dr. Kübler-Ross stages. I confirmed with the best cardiology consultative help that he could not withstand open-heart surgery for valve replacement,[32] and I made house calls on him right to the end. He received the best medicine I could prescribe, parsed out by his attentive wife, he breathed his concentrated oxygen while I kept him dried out with diuretics to relieve his struggling heart, he had regular visits from a kind and caring hospice nurse, and at the very end he died a peaceful death at home, with his wife and children at his bedside.

Missy Cartel, Margaret Bottingham, and Teresa Adams were far more challenging—they all suffered from, and eventually died from, the complications of what doctors commonly call Organic Brain Syndrome—a destruction of the brain by an autoimmune disease (MS), by a virus (Creutzfeldt-Jakob disease) or by a drug (Interferon, although the Hepatitis C may have played a role). Their planning was fundamentally the same as it is for most people who are elderly with dementia, involving drugs to keep them comfortable, not using life-saving drugs (antibiotics, etc.) near the end that would prolong their demented lives, and using nursing homes and hospice Care for the emphasis on their comfort.

Should each of us think about planning for these kinds of eventualities in our lives? Should we assume we will *not* be demented and can fend for ourselves as time passes and age becomes replaced by aged? The answer to both questions is yes, but before going out to buy long-term care policies or spending significant money for eventualities that are unlikely, the risk and the benefit probabilities need to be considered. Certainly, dementia can occur without any predisposing risk factors, but then car crashes occur, trees fall, meteors strike, and unpredictable things *actually happen*! If you are living where there is a shortage of primary care physicians (that is, more of a shortage than already exists across the country), or if your community has no decent hospital, no decent assisted care living facilities, inadequate availability of hospice nurses, or no decent nursing homes, then it might be a good idea to move if you can. It makes no sense living where there cannot be the support so often necessary, even if you think you will never need it.

The key is to ensure you have a doctor available who can help salvage your soul under these unpredictable circumstances. Furthermore, if you develop increased risks of an earlier-arriving mortality, it is important that you make early arrangements for upcoming support needs, while the family you have created and relished during your lifetime brings some cheer to the days which might otherwise become very dark and very lonely.

And, if the planning is done right, there can be some sunshine at the end. My patient of several decades, Mrs. Marcella Mander, was a slender and sweet lady of 90 who suffered from increasing complications of diverticulum problems in her intestinal system. She had abdominal pain from time to time, she had to undergo surgery for the placement of a colostomy, and with the help of a capable visiting nurse and her extraordinary daughter, and she was able to care for the maintenance of her diet and her colostomy bag. She lived alone in her beachside home, her husband having died several years before, but her son and daughter visited her on a regular basis. She lost weight and became thinner from her condition, but with a clear mind and remarkable insight, she determined that the forces were soon going to overwhelm her. When she asked me to make a house call one day, she knew it would be the final house call, and as I walked into her bedroom to greet her, with her daughter standing nearby, I was struck by two most remarkable things.

First, she was clearly septic—there was a fever controlled by Tylenol,[33] there was some abdominal discomfort controlled by powerful analgesics, but there was some systemic weakness and discomfort from the bacteria entering her bloodstream again. But much more remarkable, as a sign that Mrs. Mander clearly knew this would be my final visit to her home, she had very carefully made herself beautiful with eye shadow, lipstick, and a trace of coloring to her cheeks. Her hair was coiffed perfectly so that, even while approaching death's door, she looked as radiant as I had ever seen her in the thirty years of life that she had been under my care.

As her daughter watched, she lifted her head just an inch or two from the pillow and with a beautiful smile, she said, "Hello, Roger, it is so nice of you to stop by. I'm doing just fine, you know?"

And the next morning, she peacefully slipped away with the grace and the beauty of a woman who paid attention to planning that allowed her final days and hours to be among the best of her life.

# CHAPTER 6

## *I'm Doing the Best I Can*
## *and Other Things That May Kill You*

The emergency call from Dr. Ralph Martin came to my office that afternoon, as I awaited his report on my patient undergoing open heart surgery to replace his defective aortic heart valve. Dr. Martin was an outstanding cardiovascular surgeon who had operated on many of my patients over several years, often in a distant hospital near Los Angeles—he was well-trained, competent, and hardworking, on top of the heart surgery game and as good as they get. Our mutual patient, a very wealthy, powerful, and socially prominent 72-year-old Dexter Bradley, had undergone my usual Internal Medicine preparation for the surgery the week before, the so-called "pre-op exam," including a comprehensive physical evaluation, an electrocardiogram, a treadmill, and a battery of blood studies to confirm he was ready for surgery. I found him to be in great shape except for his failing heart valve and I handed him over to Dr. Martin for the surgery.

"Hello, Ralph, thanks for getting back to me," I said into the telephone, closing my office door and sitting down. "How did everything go?"

"Roger..." Martin said before pausing for five seconds of silence. As I waited and began to wonder if the line might have become disconnected, the surgeon started to speak again. From the quivering of his voice, I realized with some shock that Dr. Ralph Martin was struggling to bring his emotions under control...and this surgeon was not an emotional man. I felt the chill of sudden sweat as he unfolded his story.

The next five minutes of conversation took me back to an event during my previous time as a nuclear reactor operator with the crew of the fast-attack submarine, the USS Viperfish.[34] We were hundreds of feet below the surface at that time, we had just been told our mission failures had again delayed our scheduled return to Pearl Harbor after having spent innumerable weeks and more than two months suffering minor and major failures and disasters. I had joined the others with the crew to sit down for breakfast before starting another four hours on-watch at the nuclear reactor control panel in our engine room. Our morale, during this time of no measureable success while hundreds of feet under the Pacific Ocean, was terrible...about as bad as I had ever seen. Our biggest problem was that we had failed and repeatedly failed to find mission success, as everything possible on the submarine seemed to keep breaking or malfunctioning around us.

The men of the crew were quiet at the breakfast tables, almost a hostile silence, as the Cream of Wheat cereal was served with eggs and bacon on the side. I already knew that a quiet submarine crew is almost always an unhappy crew as everyone around me wanted to finish our mission, to find some increment of

91

success, to have *something* to go right for a change. We glumly spooned in the cereal as we mulled unhappy thoughts like what an incoming Soviet torpedo might sound like or how many more weeks we had before seeing sunlight.

Suddenly, one of the larger crew members, a huge machinist mate sitting near the end of the table, spewed out the cereal from his mouth on the table in front of him and hollered, "There's worms in the *!#**!@#!** cereal."

All of us immediately stopped chewing and examined the bowls of cereal in front of us. *Simultaneously*, every man in the compartment, including myself, began violently spewing cereal from our mouths on the table, complete with little swarms of very *very* tiny white worms that were still alive and had been perfectly camouflaged in the white grain of the cereal. Somehow, some insect creatures had achieved entry into the dry cereal storage container and had vigorously reproduced during the past many weeks to create a large volume of writhing worms within the container. Several of the men began vomiting while hollering for the cook, some of them using language with swear words I had never previously heard, even after five years in the Navy. Ten seconds later, the acting cook that morning, Benjamin Speeter, a small man with a gentle manner and a third class petty officer emblem clipped to his collar, rushed out of the galley to appear before us in the dining room.

He looked around with wide eyes at the men spitting more cereal onto the table and another couple of men now vigorously retching. All of us glared ferociously at the man and began to verbally roar at him with an intense message about the worm situation. The cook picked up one of the bowls still holding some uneaten cereal, he studied the cereal and the worms carefully, he winced and he looked at all of us.

He could have told us it was added protein, placed into the cereal for nutritional value. He could have tasted a sample and noted it really didn't taste all that bad, speculating how the worms survived the cooking process. He could have and should have said *anything* other than what he actually said.

Unfortunately, that was the moment that Benjamin Speeter said the worst thing possible anybody could ever say on a nuclear submarine. "Come on, you guys," he whined, "*I'm doing the best I can!*"

Everything on the submarine seemed to get worse, much worse, from that point on as more equipment failed, more critical systems malfunctioned, and our primary espionage mission remained unsuccessful. Through it all, for the remainder of the patrol, the mantra, "*I'm doing the best I can!*" could be heard over and over again, most frequently spoken loudly in the area of Benjamin who became the master of ignoring everything said in his vicinity.

"*I'm doing the best I can*" became synonymous with the best efforts being made and disastrous results following.

Three weeks later, we finally moored at Pearl Harbor and bolted from the ship for transportation to the nightspots of Waikiki, all of us wanting to have some beverages, *lots* of beverages, and blow off some steam. As far as I was aware, nobody had any adverse GI effects from the worm consumption, and after a few

93

nights in Waikiki, it might have all blown over. But, as we left the submarine, poor Benjamin Speeter decided he didn't want to be on our boat any longer and formally non-volunteered from the submarine Navy.[35] During our next patrol back at sea a few weeks later, again spending several months under the ocean thousands of miles from land, we never saw any worms again, the equipment stopped breaking or malfunctioning, we never heard the "doing the best I can" phrase from anyone, and we finally experienced a resounding mission success (to the great unhappiness of the Soviet Union).

"Roger," the surgeon haltingly said into my telephone, "I must tell you that our patient is currently brain-dead."

Frozen in my chair, I listened to his description of the saga in the distant operating room, of how the veteran respiratory therapist accidently inserted a critical one-way valve *backwards* into the tubing that fed the patient's respiratory system, blocking the anesthetized man from receiving oxygen while under anesthesia. I heard the description of the neurological changes Mr. Bradley had experienced as his brain became virtually stroked to oblivion, a massive disaster of so-called prolonged cerebral anoxia, and of how the surgeon had gone ahead and fixed the valve anyway, even knowing his patient would never awaken. I heard of the anesthesiologist and the entire surgical team trying without success to revive the patient after his surgery, and of the neurologist confirming the presence of a permanent irreversible state of brain death.

I hung up the telephone quietly, I mumbled a couple of Navy curses I remembered under my breath, and I left my office for the long drive to the hospital.

He was in the post-op intensive care unit of the hospital, lying on his back with the respirator breathing for him. His nurse glanced at me with a look of fleeting despair and rushed out of the room. I did more testing to confirm there was no brain activity in the patient who was only moving with the forced air flow from the respirator, I confirmed that his pupils were fixed and dilated, and I called his wife, who had already been informed by the surgeon. I told her I would do everything I could to keep her husband comfortable, and I braced myself for her response.

"You will ensure that your patient is dead by Thursday, Dr. Dunham," she screamed into the telephone. "I have scheduled my husband's funeral for Friday!"

"Your patient," not "my husband," she identified the brain-dead man lying in the intensive care unit, her definition now placing all responsibilities about the fate of her husband directly on my shoulders. As I returned to the waiting patients in my office and struggled to complete the day, the question kept burning through my mind. How could this happen, how could this happen? The hospital was a smaller hospital, but these surgeries had been done there before, by this surgeon, and by this group of anesthesiologists and respiratory therapists. They were all good, very good, but the surgeon was responsible for everything that happened in the operating room, being the "captain" of the operating team, and so of course the surgeon was accountable for the mistake.

understanding.  That crash killed three young Chinese girls and severely injured 187 others.

As it is with pilots, is it the same with hospital teams and hospitals?  If experience is so important, especially *recent* experience above and beyond that required for certification, shouldn't that play a profound role for hospitals, surgeons, surgical teams, and physicians in general?  But, do we as patients look at this critical factor with the hope and the faith that everybody will do well because they certainly will be doing the best they can?

The ultimate question for us to ask, then, before a scheduled operation with a certified team of specialists, is how many of these surgeries have been done in our chosen hospital, and how many of these surgeries by this team have been performed *recently*, like, in the past six months?  Furthermore, from Dexter Bradley's case, how many of these kinds of surgeries were performed in this small hospital, its very size alone suggesting not enough?  All too often, we assume that we'll be fine because this seems to be such a nice hospital, we trust the surgeon, the people are all so friendly, or the surgical team has such a good reputation.

If all this is true, if experience is so profoundly important, could it be expected that teams and hospitals performing fewer operations per year would have higher risks of complications or death from the surgery?  If surgery is to be performed to *lower* the risks of mortality for a patient and to delay the probability of death, as was the case with Dexter Bradley, wouldn't it be a good idea to have the surgery performed by a surgical team and in a hospital, like our local hospital, where similar surgery is done several times a day, perhaps hundreds of times per year? If the problem is that, in spite of competent physicians and therapists in a low-volume hospital, everybody *doing the best they can*, would the results and the mortality be lower at higher volume hospitals? Or, to put it another way, do low-volume hospitals have too many tiny worms in their cereals?

The answer in many cases is yes.

Numerous studies confirm this, dating back all the way to the 1970's when the outcomes of surgery in general were studied. In one early study of that decade,[36] if surgeries were done in hospitals that performed more than 200 surgical procedures in the year, there were 25%-41% fewer patient deaths than in lower-volume hospitals. In our community, at Dexter Bradley's hospital, in fact, the operating teams there did less than 50 of these procedures per year, a low-volume track record by any measurement. After Mr. Bradley's sudden accelerated mortality and death, (in spite of a successful valve replacement), the cardiac program at that hospital was closed down and all further such operations were performed at a higher-volume hospital several miles away.

Looking below the surface of the numbers, it is clear that mistakes happen because of the "human factor," that allows mistakes, oversights, or lapses, when the volume of procedures is not adequate. Why would smaller hospitals with low-volume procedures even consider performing these surgeries when the outcomes are more likely to accelerate mortality? The answer is that they do so only partly for the convenience for the patient; it turns out that, not surprisingly, money also plays a role. A more recent review[37] looked at Medicare's financial incentives for smaller hospitals to allow certain orthopedic procedures. It was found that there is, in fact, an increased reimbursement from Medicare to these hospitals (apparently, to keep smaller hospitals afloat) even though the mortality rate in the smaller hospitals are nearly twice that of larger hospitals.

Examples abound. With cancer surgery, for example, it was found[38] that the mortality of patients having their esophagus removed for cancer treatment at high-volume hospitals was 3%, compared with 17% at low-volume hospitals. Although efforts have been made to shift challenging surgeries to high-volume hospitals, and to publish mortality data for physicians, there has been fierce resistance by the hospitals and by the surgeons, for obvious reasons. The best advice, then, for a reduction of your own personal mortality risks, if surgery emerges in your future, is to *politely* ask your surgeon how many of the anticipated surgeries he or she has done in the past year, and how many such surgeries are performed at the chosen hospital. The results of such questions, if acted upon, will likely improve your own mortality risks and the chances of survival at least until another day.

What about the consideration that it would be good to put out the fire of emerging disease before it has barely started? If there is a risk of accelerated mortality and an earlier death from something like cancer, why not find the cancer in the early stages before it begins to spread, before a major surgery is even needed? Wouldn't it make sense to avoid bigger or more complicated surgery in large or small hospitals by finding problems such as cancer before much growth occurs? This is being done to some extent by genetic studies that correlate a specific set of genes with increased risks, most prominently in the breast cancer arena, with mammograms supplementing the picture. But what about a wide-area CT scan from time to time, searching for the tiny cancer that would otherwise escape detection? Seems like a good idea, but as with everything in the world of biology, the answer is not simple.

Not too many years ago, standalone radiology centers and others began offering "total body scans" as a part of an effort to prove there was no underlying hidden disease that might generate increased risks of an accelerated mortality. There were even "Valentine Day Specials" with loved ones offered an opportunity to get their scans at a reduced price—truly an element of hucksterism unfit for professionals in medicine. These CT scans were the standard rotating X-ray scans, looking for abnormalities as small as a grain of rice.

The ads from these centers can be persuasive, such as the following on-line announcement from a California radiology center:

-*The $425 Full Body Scan includes a comprehensive study of major internal organs from the neck (thyroid) to the hips (pelvis).*
-*The exam is fast, noninvasive, and comfortable, with less than a minute of actual scan time*
-*Included in the price is the Heart Scan, Lung Scan, Body Scan, and a Report by our Board-Certified Radiologist*
-*Also included with every Full Body Scan is a personal and confidential consultation with one of our*

*physicians so you can understand your findings and ask any questions you may have (the consultation will consist of either a telephone consult or a 10-15 minute discussion).*
*-A Head Scan can be added for only an additional $50.*

The problems with all this promotion, and what the ads don't mention, is:

- The significant amount of radiation delivered to the patient with each scan
- The probability of false positives which may lead to many subsequent problems

The radiation issue does not show up in the ads for the scans, and yet the level of absorbed radiation from these "searching for disease" studies is significant. While a chest X-ray delivers about 2-10 mrem[39] of gamma energy, and a mammogram delivers about 20-70 mrem, the dose for a whole-body scan is much higher. Dr. Thomas Shope, a special assistant at the FDA's Center for Devices and Radiological Health, advised a Federal Drug Administration panel reviewing this issue that the average whole-body CT scan delivered from 200 mrem to as much as 2,000 mrem.[40] Furthermore, American College of Radiology (ACR) took the position,[41] nearly fifteen years ago that "there is no evidence that total-body CT screening is cost-effective or is effective in prolonging life. In addition, the ACR is concerned that this procedure will lead to the discovery of numerous findings that will not ultimately affect patients' health, but will result in increased patient anxiety, unnecessary follow-up examinations and treatments, and wasted expense."

What about just scanning the chest, looking into the lungs for abnormalities ranging from cancers to early tuberculosis? Or scanning the heart to determine the "Calcium Index Score" in an effort to predict the probability of a heart attack? Listening to the proponents of such scans, it would seem that you could just about scan anything to find anything and all of it will help lower mortality from a myriad of diseases. However, just scanning the chest alone can deliver as much as 1600 mrem of radiation[42]--and amazingly, this is more, much more, than I used to receive in a year (by radiation film badge measurements) as a reactor operator on our submarine with neutron and gamma radiation from nuclear reactor power settings often running as high as 100%.[43] Even though this medical radiation concern is now improving across the United States with enhanced techniques, the use of any of these scans, (including those that measure calcium buildup in heart arteries or the follow-up enhanced heart arterial studies to measure obstruction) is a process still seeking its proper place in the diagnostic armamentarium of this country.

Regarding the probability of false-positive scans that result in fear and dangers from unneeded follow-up procedures, more questions plague the medical industry. Questions needing answers relate to the scans being done in patients who have no symptoms, versus being done in patients with significant symptoms or findings such as chest pain, weight loss, or lymph node enlargement. Furthermore, the *results* of the scan are important—if the scan is a false positive (showing something that later turns out to be nothing important), it may take biopsies to rule out actual disease. Biopsies are expensive and create risks for patients, and depending on what part of the body is being biopsied, the biopsy procedure could lead to complications and even death. This is particularly important in CT scans of the brain, where a benign growth such as a meningioma may be stable for decades; follow-up CT scans, then, may be needed to prove a stable abnormality, delivering more radiation, again, which carries a (small) degree of necessary risk.

All this is why it is a bad idea for people to independently listen to ads and then run out and start getting scans and studies offered by various profit-seeking entities without thoughtful input by physicians (who, importantly, are not connected with any of these facilities). With good medical input from your personal physician, the proper balance between the cost of studies, the amount of radiation, the probability of false positives, the genetic susceptibility, the age of a patient, symptoms or lack of symptoms, findings on physical examination, family history, etc., can all be put together to develop the best plan for the future. If this kind of detailed thinking is not applied, the probability of a useful course of action becomes rapidly and drastically reduced, and the probable outcome then is a waste of money and time, the adverse consequences of a biopsy that might not have been needed, or the cumulative effects of radiation on a sensitive body as the years go by.

I learned the shocking reality about the finality of death before I even became a medical student, during the grinding year of premed studies at the University of Southern California, when I elected to watch autopsies at the Los Angeles County Hospital department of pathology. The plan was to learn some human anatomy by direct observation of anatomy.

When I first walked in the autopsy room that morning, with Grant's Atlas of Anatomy tucked under my arm, the jolt beyond the powerful formaldehyde odor and beyond the rows of bodies being disassembled in a remarkably thorough manner by the pathologists was the coming face-to-face with the absolute irreversible finality of death. The bodies of those men and those women lying on the tables had all been recently alive, going to their doctors in some cases, assaulted by violent criminals in others, struck down on the freeway in yet others, all of them brought to their ends in a manner that was, for most of them, entirely unsuspected. Given a chance to change the circumstances of their death would have prevented many of their deaths by the most miniscule change in activity during the final minutes or hour. A changed route on the road or sidewalk, a decision not to have surgery or not to take a powerful legal or illegal drug, making changes in association with certain friends, or a change in the element of trust placed in somebody who seemed to be doing the best they could, all could have prevented their body's presence that first morning on those cold stainless steel autopsy tables. For each of them, no further decisions would be made, and nothing was awaited but a formal physician report identifying altered tissues and toxicities. Burned into my mind for my entire career in medicine, then, was that everything there in that room underscored the importance of identifying the elements of mortality before death and then making the right decisions to prevent the death. This meant not just doing the best I could during the years ahead but also actually preventing the death that would otherwise overtake the patient.

For my very sweet patient, Mrs. Sutter, a 57-year-old woman with fluid in her right lung cavity, it was with complete innocence that she agreed to my request for a needle to be inserted into her chest by the competent pulmonary specialist, the needle was to withdraw a couple of liters of fluid to expand her lung and to provide us with a diagnosis. But the needle struck a blood vessel, an aberrant blood vessel that usually would not have been there, the subsequent rapid bleeding dropped her blood pressure, and in spite of the urgent transfer to the Intensive Care Unit and the administration of fluids and plasma and everything else everyone could think of, she suffered a massive stroke and became vegetative before her final escort to the hereafter in the arms of Morpheus several weeks later.

Everybody did the best they could for Mrs. Sutter, both before and after the needle created the internal bleeding state of havoc. This was not malpractice, and even her poor grown son was accepting of her fate and the final outcome. It was one of those small potential risks listed on the consent form, like it had been on consent forms for so many people who lie on the autopsy table at the LA County Medical Center. As terrible as everyone felt, the fluid analysis did reveal a diagnosis of cardiovascular disease predicting a downward spiral into weeks or months of suffering if the needle had *not* been inserted, none of which gave me comfort.

Other cases may not be so reassuring about alternative pathways. During my years at the UCLA School of Medicine, a senior physician guiding the students to know and learn more, told us of his mother.

She was a 74-year-old woman, who had suffered from a bowel malfunction creating progressively severe weight loss. Because of her age and the cachexia she suffered, her doctors had felt surgery was inadvisable and had elected to allow the yet-to-be-identified malignancy to carry her on to the state of weakness, continued bed rest, and finally with the help of a hospice nurse, to the eventual end of her life. His mother, the physician told us, had died a fairly comfortable death and he was happy for that, but after she died, he felt she still deserve a firm final diagnosis, now that the abdominal problem could be easily determined on the autopsy table.

The pathologist made the large abdominal incision that would reveal the problem; he aimed the light directly into the depths of her abdomen, and did not need the subsequent positive microscopic and culture information to confirm that the doctor's mother had been suffering from gastrointestinal tuberculosis. Her TB skin test had been negative, [44] and this disease had never been identified as she traveled down the road to what had seemed to be an inevitable death. In fact, the condition would have been easily treatable with appropriate anti-TB pills earlier in the disease and his mother certainly should have had another fifteen to twenty good years ahead; the senior doctor told us the story in a quiet and humbled voice, underscoring his continuing sadness that she had found mortality and death years before her time from something unsuspected as everybody around her was doing the best they could.

This lady's case underscored a single sentence from one of the brightest pathologists who lectured our medical school class at UCLA. "Whole herds of physicians will join in the increasingly certain diagnostic stampede," he told us during a lecture on infectious diseases. "And as more physicians join in, they will move down the road that gives an increasingly smooth ride, paved with the golden *collective certainty* of the diagnosis, right up to the point where the scalpel of the pathologist proves them all wrong." And so this doctor who lost his mother to a treatable disease, speaking quietly to our small group of riveted medical students, told us without resentment or recriminations to always doubt our diagnoses and to always seek a rock-solid certainty that may alter the course of treatment and save lives. The translation of this concept is that, if a physician you have chosen to oversee your diagnostic elements of healthcare seems to be brash and confident of his path, be wary, you need a physician who will work to the end of this earth to be as correct as is scientifically possible, to confirm the right diagnosis before the wrong diagnosis may result in the patient's death.

This element of humility was not on the surface of my mind when Mr. George Stanton appeared in my office one day with a cough and slight discomfort in his right shoulder. He was a nonsmoker and so even before his examination, I presumed the man had bronchitis of some kind. I thumped on his lungs to ensure there was no fluid, I listened carefully to ensure there was no noise of a pneumonia, and considering the fact of the cough being dry, that he had no weight loss, that he had no chest pain, and that there was no fever, I elected to not give him any antibiotics and sent him home with instructions to take some prescription cough medicine.

"It's probably a viral bronchitis, antibiotics usually don't help," I told him as he moved his right shoulder around, smiled, and asked if I had anything for the arthritis in his shoulder. Four days later, George called and informed me that the dry cough was continuing and didn't seem to be going away. No, he was not coughing up any blood or bringing up any significant sputum, and yes, the ibuprofen seemed to help his left shoulder, thank you, doctor, he told me. Since he was anxious about the cough, and possibly an early bacterial problem had emerged, I prescribed a broad-spectrum antibiotic for the next four days. Five days later, with no improvement, he was back in my office again for reexamination.

I examined him again and discovered a miniscule degree of swelling of his right arm that he stated had just started, causing a tightening of his ring on his right hand.

"Do I need a chest X-ray?" he asked.

"George, you will need chest X-ray, but you also will need some blood studies and you need a CT scan of your chest," I told him, "and we need to schedule all of this ASAP." Within the next twenty-four hours, he was in the hospital; the mass in his right upper lung had been identified along with a lymph node above his right collarbone. The lymph node was promptly biopsied and we confirmed the microscopic and clinical diagnosis of an acute lymphoma malignancy with swelling from pressure on the vein draining his right arm. In the hands of an excellent oncologist, intravenous administration of multiple anti-lymphoma medications moved him in the direction of a potential cure.

After decades of treating viral bronchitis, and occasionally bacterial bronchitis and pneumonia, a man with a malignant lymphoma walks into my office with a cough. Is there room for humility, for doubt in my diagnosis, and should I get a chest X-ray on *every* patient with a cough? If there is anything to be learned from this, by both the physician as well as the patient, it is that the physician's work for a patient is a *practice* of medicine, with large quantities of doubt, and large efforts to seek the truth without over-treating and over-medicating. Where the line is drawn in this profoundly variable spectrum of disease and patient circumstance is always the challenge....

# CHAPTER 7
## What would God say?

Ronald Blackburn's paramedic ambulance screamed into the Catholic hospital emergency room at about 8 PM and was immediately followed by his distraught and aging wife, Betty. Blackburn was an elderly man approaching 90 years and he was in a desperate condition, in an ominous state of shock from a profoundly low blood pressure as the ruptured aneurysm in his abdomen rapidly bled into his body. The team of emergency room physicians ripped the chain holding a tiny Hamsa[45] from his chest and worked furiously on him as the hospital staff escorted his wife to the nearby waiting room. Over the next half hour, she repeatedly asked if she could talk with the ER physician but was told the doctor was still with her husband and that he would soon give her an update.

When Dr. Salgundi finally entered the waiting room, he was accompanied by one of the hospital's Catholic sisters, and after handing the broken Hamsa piece of jewelry to Mrs. Blackburn, he gently advised her that her husband could not be saved in spite of the sustained and heroic efforts to stabilize him for emergency surgery. When she asked if she could see him, she was told they were "straightening him up" but that she could see him in about fifteen minutes. Dr. Salgundi then asked if she would like to talk with a priest, a minister, or perhaps a rabbi. She thought for a moment and then shook her head, saying, "That won't be necessary." The physician then spoke some kind condolences and finally departed the room, leaving the Catholic sister and Mrs. Blackburn together for about five minutes of discussion. By the time I arrived from my home, the sister had departed and Mrs. Blackburn was sitting alone in the waiting room, her hands clutched tightly together.

"Betty," I said, walking into the room, "I just spoke with the emergency room doctor and I am so sorry that they could not save Ron." I reached out to take her hand and added, "It sounded like they did everything they could to save him, his aorta just ruptured…."

The woman stood up furiously and glared at me. She would not take my hand and her eyes burned with rage as she said, "That sister or that nun, or whatever you call them, just talked with me. She said that God is good! Why do they say that God is good? *At a time like this*? What does that mean, why would they say that? God is not good when my husband has been ripped away from me and is now lying on a table, DEAD!"

I looked at her for a moment as she suffered her anguish, considering what I could possibly say. The comments from the Catholic sister had been well meaning, I knew, reflecting the religious belief of a merciful God who could be benevolent under the proper circumstances. Ronald was Mrs. Blackburn's third husband, but they had been happily married for about 20 years, she had prepared their dinner that night, and as he had stood up to wash the dishes, he had suddenly doubled over with severe pain in his abdomen.

And, twenty-five minutes later, Ronald Blackburn was dead.

We sat down and I talked with her, clarifying that the Catholic sister was just trying to reassure her that a God that was good and who would certainly see that the man belonged in heaven would salvage her husband's soul. She clearly had misinterpreted the session with the nun, feeling she had been told that God was good in taking him away from her, leaving her alone in the world, causing her anger in that time of her great emotional suffering. We talked about what a good man her husband had been, what a good life he had led, and how lucky he was to have had such a good wife. She became more settled and peaceful, I finally led her into the emergency room and to the curtains surrounding the body of her husband to say a final goodbye before she left to stay with a relative that night.

I never did ask her what her religion was, but as our discussion continued, it was quite clear that she held strong Christian beliefs. We had talked about God judging her husband favorably, we had talked about heaven, and we did discuss the "hereafter." However, I'm just a doctor and with her tears, her anger, and her need for some helpful thoughts, there I was, talking about religion, a subject not included much in my experience or in my decade of training. In that little waiting room, her dead husband lying nearby on his gurney, Mrs. Blackburn and I had the most powerful stimulus for establishing some kind of religious understanding, something, *anything*, to bridge our daily life with the reality of death…not just for her husband but for ourselves as well.

There is almost a reverse relationship between age and religion—in younger people, mortality is largely an abstraction (unless nature or accidents intervene), but as we all age, mortality begins to stare us in the face along with the inevitable link with *what happens to us after we die*? This can't be the end, when our eyes close, when our heart beats its final beat and our minds fade away…can it? No it can't, we must tell ourselves, since otherwise, what is the point of the years of our lives, why have we existed on this planet? Are we to have lived and then to be gone into nothingness?

Unacceptable, and if that is not reality for you now, hang on, because as the years go by….

The real question must be asked, where is the concept of religion, the primary purpose that seems to explain the "hereafter," in the United States and in the world today? Furthermore, is there *more* religion, or *less*? There are five main religions in the world today, Hinduism, Buddhism, Judaism, Islam, and Christianity, and in spite of the horrific battles between the faithful in each religion over thousands of years, right up to today and certainly into the future, they are all unified by teaching how a good life today affects the fate of the "soul" in the hereafter. They do this through the preaching of individual leaders (Jesus Christ, Mohammed, Buddha or Moses), by historical precedent, or by traditions written in the millions of pages outlining specific religious elements carried to the faithful by rabbis, priests, ministers, Da'ees[46] and others.

Ronald Blackburn had died a rapid and terribly painful death and there was a high statistical probability (although I never asked) that he was a Christian, that is, that he believed in the teachings of Jesus Christ or that at least he was a follower of Christ to whatever extent he felt was appropriate. The term Christian is derived from the Greek word *christianos*, which is in turn, derived from the word *Christos* or Christ, meaning, "anointed one." In the realm of Christianity (70% of the United States population), Americans in the Catholic Church remain prominent, comprising about 20% of the country's population while Protestants comprise about 45%. The Catholic's resoundingly positive view of death for those who have led a "good life" reflects the faithful's Christian view of the *afterlife* in heaven, the final reward for having lived a good life.

As the chief of the hospital's medical staff at that time, I had visited the sisters' "Mother House" in Illinois a few months earlier, and I had been impressed by the peaceful and powerful faith that permeated the environment around the many Catholic sisters living there. This had balanced my previous guarded opinion, fostered by my early years, in the third grade, where the Catholic teachers had battered me about, generally using their rulers upon my head to enforce classroom policies. In retrospect, much of the smacking was well deserved, considering my generally turbulent behavior patterns at that time. However, after numerous confessions to the priest didn't seem to help my circumstances, I finally blew out all the candles in the church next to the elementary school. Caught in the act, several Catholic sisters chased me out of the church and up the street, waving their rulers and creating a genuine fear of God in me before I escaped and mercifully the next day became a Protestant for the remainder of my life. Although I am sure I had nothing to do with it, unfortunately for the Catholic Church, the number of Catholic elementary schools in the United States has drastically declined, recently noted to have dropped from more than 10,000 when I was being smacked about, to about 5,000 during the passing of about 50 years.[47]

But the Mother House taught me the strength of belief brought about by a lifetime of religion, unfortunately not communicated effectively to Mrs. Blackburn who would have been impressed by the nun's dedication to help suffering patients and their relatives, a process that was emblematic for the sisters in this Catholic hospital. At the Mother House, there was a large highly polished board across one of the walls, with about two hundred golden plaques carrying the name of sisters who had expired during the previous decades. The Mother Superior there (fortunately unaware of my abysmal early elementary school history) told me the sisters in the faith were greatly looking forward to their futures in heaven, bolstered by the solid belief that an eternity of goodness and contentment awaited them. The sisters of the Catholic Church were, therefore, *actually looking forward to death*, a faith-driven concept that I noted in my Catholic Nun patients I cared for as they entered their own arenas of mortality.

Heaven, envisioned as somewhere up in the sky, is worth thinking about, since it is the cornerstone of the Christianity reward, relating to sins, forgiveness, and the compassion of Christ and of God, all of which plays a role in providing an improved chance of a pleasant existence after death. Furthermore, since there is only one alternative to heaven (at least in the Christian faith) and nothing in between heaven and the purgatory below, heaven is clearly worthy of strong consideration, especially if the "Judgment Day" is suddenly roaring into our lives. "Doing good things so that you may go to heaven" is not seen negatively in the Christian faith, since the fact of "doing good things" is measured in its own right irrespective of an awaiting reward. This pathway of goodness, defined as the way shown by Christ, is a part of virtually all subsets of Christianity, leading to a huge range of practices within each of these religious systems with many different peripheral beliefs. There are no fewer than 15 of these systems within the realm of Christianity, from Catholics to Presbyterians, to Lutherans, Methodists, Mormons, Baptists, Christian Scientists, and so on.

Heaven, the centerpiece of it all, is most simply defined[48] as "the place, often considered very pleasant or good, where God lives and where good people go after they die." As simple as this sounds, the methodology by which somebody can get there is what adds to the challenges of experiencing a worsening medical condition with mortality beginning to loom ahead. If you have been a sinner, the prospects for heaven are diminished; if you have committed any one of several "mortal sins[49]," your chances of heaven are nearly zero unless there is a fulfillment of "penance" without which you will likely be damned to hell.

For Mr. Blackburn, doubled over in pain from his acute and lethal bleeding problem, the issue of his impending arrival into the hereafter was not likely at the top of his mind. He didn't ask for a minister or a priest as he became incapacitated with severe pain, he didn't even ask for a doctor. He hollered for his wife to call 911 and shortly thereafter, he became unconscious, after which it would have been difficult for him to think good thoughts, to confess the sins of his life, or to request forgiveness from the highest available religious authorities to be found in the hospital.

If his religion had mandated he undergo baptism, earlier in life, his chances of salvation at the moment of his unfortunate death might have been enhanced. However, the process of baptism, where holy water is sprinkled on one's head or the body is totally immersed in holy water, is not seen by some Christians (such as the Baptists wing of Christianity) to be useful for salvation, but more of an act of Christian obedience...a good thing, however, to improve the odds of reaching heaven. Furthermore, even if Mr. Blackburn had been baptized as a child and then had committed one of the mortal sins thereafter, he would have been banished from religious protection and sent directly to hell unless he underwent a lengthy and arduous public penance. Because of this risk, many people with religious convictions may delay baptism until later adult life, rather than as a child, to lessen the risks of this banishment process should a mortal sin occur during youth. However, if Ronald Blackburn had needed baptism at the conclusion of his dinner, or if public penance had been on his menu, it would have been too late.

In the early days of my medical practice, the death of Mrs. Esther Silverstein burned into my mind for two unexpected and remarkable reasons. A pleasant and mildly obese 53-year-old woman, she had been brought to the hospital with chest pain that resolved after her cardiac studies showed minimal heart damage. Recovering in a private room a few days later, she had suddenly hollered that a crushing chest pain had just developed, and within just a few seconds, she suffered a complete cardiac arrest. Working at the nursing station nearby, I raced into the room to answer the hospital's "Code Blue" call and spent the next hour providing chest compressions as the respiratory therapist pumped oxygen into her lungs. We tried, we did everything I had ever learned in the years of my training during that hour, but even though her eyes opened and she watched me with terror as I continued chest compressions, and even though we performed direct cardiac injections, defibrillation shocks, and intravenous infusions of numerous medications, there was no change in her heart's ability to generate pressure and pump adequately.

I finally turned to the therapist and reluctantly asked, "How long have we been doing this?"

He checked the clock and announced, "It's been well over an hour, doc."

With a finality that confirmed my thoughts that I had done everything possible, I announced to the room packed with medical personnel, "Let's call it."

But, before I could move from her body and step off the bed, to my horror, I saw Esther Silverstein's arms suddenly reach straight up above her body in a horrific conscious movement, as if she was imploring me, *begging me*, to continue with the now-futile effort. Her blood pressure, which had been kept marginally adequate from the chest compressions, then plummeted to zero, her eyes then rapidly glazed over and closed, and her arms dropped to the bed to complete her final movements in death.

After a moment of absolute silence, the nurses began the grim task of making her body look presentable for the family now waiting down the hall. When their work was completed and Mrs. Silverstein *almost* looked like she was sleeping, I brought the five family members into the room, her husband and several children with their spouses moving single-file, their tear-streaked faces already filled with grief. They saw her body and a quiet murmuring filled the room as they began to pray. They quickly opened every window in the room and sat down in chairs as they finished their prayers. I tried to console them as my mind attempted to block out the pleading arms held up by the woman in her last seconds of life, the movements reflecting that her mind and her entire being were begging for the imminent mortality not to become her reality.

And then, after having witnessed a woman begging for a life that was no more, the second calamity of the day occurred. In the silence of the room as my condolences ended and I finished saying what I could to ease the suffering in the sad gathering of loved ones, I reached over to the bed and slowly pulled the sheets up from her chest to cover her face. To this day, I do not know why I did that except that I had seen it done before as a kind of respect for some privacy for the recently deceased. Also, somewhere in the back of my mind, I recalled all the television programs and movies I had seen showing the deceased being covered with a sheet, wrapped up in various ways, or placed in a "body bag" for presumably the same reason.

The reaction of the family to my covering her face was immediate and intense. There was a gasp from several of the relatives, the husband stood up and reached over, and with a quick movement, brought the sheet back down to her chest. "Doctor," he said, staring at me with anger, "we will take care of everything from this point on."

I tried to apologize, saying that I meant no disrespect, and his eyes finally softened as he led me from the room. In the corner of the hall, away from the relatives and hospital workers, he began speaking with intensity about the rituals of the Jewish families after the death of a family member. His wrinkled eyes watched me closely as he spoke, his weathered face showing no emotion, his voice firm and strong.

"We are a Jewish family, doctor," he said, "and we have traditions of respect for those who have died. I understand that you are a new doctor in our community, but you must learn the ways of our faith for you will see this again. Although many families no longer follow strict practices of Jewish tradition,[50] this family does and my children closely adhere to the religious elements established during the past 4,000 years."

"I am sorry…." I started.

He held up his hand, silencing me. "You did not know, we do not blame you. However, the closing of my wife's eyes and the covering of her eyes is particularly important…it is the sacred duty of Haviv," he gestured to the room, "our first-born son, in there now with Esther. It is his duty, it is not your duty."

I nodded and he continued.

"This closing of the eyes ritual has been done for thousands of years, and after the mortician takes her away, we will prepare for her funeral."

I put my hand on his shoulder. "These elements were never discussed during the years of my…."

"Nor *should* this be a part of your medical training, doctor, for as you care for the living, we will care for the people we love who have departed." He paused, seeming to be trying to hold his emotions tightly within. "Those of our faith know about death, and we would like to sustain our traditions of respect when so often in the past this has not been the case."

And so, that morning, I learned of the traditions not just from her husband and her son, but also from the Jewish undertaker who educated me about beliefs relating to what God expects from a Jewish family for their deceased. I learned of the funerals, of the mandatory attendance of a loved one, at all times, at the side of Mrs. Silverstein reinforcing the belief that those who have died must never be left alone. I learned that the dying body, *even after death*, is to be considered a living being in all respects.[51]

And I learned about the eyes…. I learned of the traditions that direct the son (or more recently any of the children), to place broken shards of pottery, or other elements of earth, against the closed eyes of the departed person at the time of the funeral--*pottery from the earth to the eyes as the body will be returned to the earth.*

Finally, I learned that many of the stricter traditions such as the cleansing of the body, the laying of the body on the floor with lit candles placed alongside have faded over the years.[52]

And, I learned of the Torah and the effect of its teachings on Mrs. Silverstein as she had rested in the hospital bed the past couple of days, contemplating her near-mortality after her first and mild heart attack. I asked her husband about the Torah potentially giving guidance to her before she had died, as I tried to recall everything, *anything*, I had ever heard of throughout my lifetime about the Jewish religion. Her husband explained that the Torah from Moses does not provide much guidance about heaven or hell for the Jewish individual who may be entering an accelerated mortality and preparing for the hereafter. Its primary focus is a guide to following a good life right now and not what happens after death.

The body will return to the ground,[53] he told me—that is a certainty—but the soul of those who have not lived good lives might experience a hell of sorts, possibly characterized by shame and anguish at having wasted the chance to serve God. This grim thought may have served to actually calm Mrs. Silverstein as she mulled her good and productive life during her approach to the gates of death; however, if she had lived a righteous life *for the sake of an awaited heavenly reward*, she would be disrespected as making such efforts for an ulterior motive. In other words, for the now-departed Mrs. Silverstein or for any Jew who is looking at his or her arrival of mortality, the use of faith as a *means* to a favorable end, rather than something that simply creates a good life, is a strong cause for disapproval.

However, since the time of Moses, as rabbis evolved to speak the Word from this great religious figure, two distinct favorable concepts of heaven evolved: The immortal soul of Mrs. Silverstein would have a chance to "return to God," or alternatively, her soul may undergo resurrection. Although the resurrection of Christ is the basis of the Christian religion, in Judaism, resurrection may happen to an individual of the Jewish faith for the purpose of mending the world.[54] Some people with the Jewish faith, including the Silverstein family, feel that reincarnation might have been seen as a routine process, while others believe that it only occurs in unusual circumstances, and only if her soul left unfinished business behind. For this woman, facing the approach of mortality and the imminence of death, what is there ahead, a return to God or a resurrection?

And her husband, in his time of grief, took the time to bring me an understanding about what lay in store for the body of his wife of more than twenty-five years. Near the time of her death, should it be from any of the more painful curses from nature, the Jewish faith does allow the avoidance of prolonging pain (morphine?) if death is imminent and there is painful suffering; however, it does specifically prohibit euthanasia, suicide and assisted suicide as may be offered in Oregon and California. An autopsy is discouraged by the faith for Mrs. Silverstein as desecration of her body, but may be permitted to a minimal extent if required by law or if the information might save somebody's life. The individual sitting with the body may not eat or drink; also, open caskets at a funeral are strictly prohibited, there can be no embalming and there may be no cremation of the body.[55]

By the time I had washed my hands and left the hospital to begin seeing patients in my office, I had completed a brief indoctrination about poor Mrs. Silverstein and her brief couple of days to think about her future before the actual cataclysmic arrival of her mortality. I tried to bring it together in my mind, to come to conclusions that would allow me to move on. The attitude of life after death for her could be expressed as follows: For the future is inscrutable, and the accepted sources of knowledge, whether experience, or reason, or revelation, offer no clear guidance about what is to come. The only certainty is that a person must die - beyond that we can only guess. And so, when all is said and done, only one great truth about the potential for moving to God, or perhaps to a resurrection, emerges for patients like Mrs. Silverstein: God only knows.

Religions of virtually all faiths do this same kind of thing to one extent or another. They replace the fear of death that is so natural for so many of us with the belief that a good hereafter is waiting for each of us. This fundamental fear of death, which is mostly *the fear of the unknown,* is often replaced with the known goodness of a promise to heaven, or possibly a promise to be resurrected (where the human stays as a human) or to reincarnate (rebirth into a new form of existence that may be totally different[56] from the first form of existence)—if certain specifics of behavior were met while on earth. With all these people looking to meet "certain specifics of behavior" while on earth, that is to be a good person, it is natural to assume our world is a better place because of religion.

Looking at today's world, if the single concept of *tolerance* was made the cornerstone of all religions, the centuries of religious domination and oppression might, thank God, come to an end.

To understand completely how different religions of the world might view death would take a lifetime of study to just touch on the endless variables. But, almost as a source of instruction, it is valuable to observe how people like Mr. Blackburn or Mrs. Silverstein might look at what awaits them as they lay there, suffering in their hospital beds.

And so, after watching Mr. Blackburn's rapid transition into the hereafter, and after the two shocking events as Mrs. Silverstein died, the question arises, what is the role of religion in medicine, especially when the moment of emerging mortality descends into an otherwise healthy life? When a human being is suddenly facing an almost certain mortality, there is often not much time for the acquisition of religion; however a previously established religious belief within the mind of the suffering patient, if it is strong enough, can reduce, modify, or even eliminate pain and it may substantially reduce fear.

Ronald Blackburn, however, did not have a powerful religious state of mind to protect him from the fireball of pain centered in his abdomen, and his salvation came with his rapid movement into a comatose state from his low blood pressure. Esther Silverstein had a couple of days after her first heart attack to contemplate, with her family, the elements of Judaism which could protect her or perhaps modify the final crushing chest pain that escorted her in the tortures of her mortality process.

Looking at all the challenges of mortality, moving beyond the fear of the unknown, it is the pain associated with death that often creates such misery near the end. Religion has the potential to create modifications in the perception of pain by providing a relief from fear of the unknown.

Albert Schweitzer once famously said, "Pain is a more terrible lord of mankind than even death itself,"[57] and from all that I've seen during the years of my practice, he is correct. Looking at cancer alone, 30-40% of those suffering with this spectrum of disease have significant pain throughout the progression of the disease, and 65-85% of persons with advanced cancer suffer severe pain.[58] Also, half of seriously ill children suffer pain, and 20% of them have moderate to severe pain; among elders living in the community, up to half suffer significant pain problems, and this increases up to 80% of elders living in institutions, such as nursing homes, a figure representing an increasingly sizeable portion of the elderly United States population. As it is with many of the religions of the world, bringing the security of a favorable afterlife to people suffering from their individual medical disasters, promotes the concept that there could be a peacefulness (with the relief of pain) when the final stage of mortality arrives. All major religions look to direct our lives with guidelines regarding what is a good life and what isn't which has a direct relationship with a modification or termination of pain. They all do it somewhat differently (albeit with many similarities), and they look at the future after mortality has passed and death has arrived with remarkably different visions.

Before this medical disaster reached its final conclusion for Mr. Blackburn, there was this issue of the terrible excruciating pain from his ruptured abdominal aorta. Before the coma arrived, perhaps displacing some or all of the pain, the focus on his religion and the awaiting afterlife might have helped. In fact, one of the best religious examples of an effective pain-displacement phenomenon is found in a small subset of the Muslim faith, where those of the Shia denomination (about 15% of the Muslim population in the world) mark a holiday known as "Ashura"[59] by self-flagellation rituals, where the Shia Muslims (including children) use swords, spears, or a chain with blades to ritually punish and damage their bodies with remarkable tolerance of pain.[60]

During his time of suffering, as is often the case with medical conditions creating mortality, if Mr. Blackburn's mind was focused on heaven or other religious rewards, there may have been a remarkable relief from pain. This is the prize that potentially awaits those of great faith at the end, allowing a tolerance of pain approaching that seen after great trauma (such as after an automobile crash) with devastating injuries where it is observed there is minimal or no pain. Also, for human beings, understanding much of the biological basis behind pain relief has always been a medical challenge...not only because of the variance in levels of pain from similar injuries in different people (some people have a so-called "high pain threshold"), but also because the mind can seemingly displace pain under certain circumstances including great religious concentration.

With and without religion, there is not much protection from the myriad of natural elements, from abdominal disasters to cardiac coronary blockades that create severe pain. A dreaming state is of no help, if sleep could occur under such circumstances, with dreams, we can feel pain and it often may awaken us. In a coma, however, as with general anesthesia, there is no pain when everything should be painfully tearing us apart. Finally, as our bodies approach a dying state, we regularly may rely on a coma caused by uremia (a buildup of the metabolite urea resulting from failing kidneys during dehydration) to protect us from pain and suffering.

Another manipulation of the mind, hypnosis, can modify pain in cancer and multiple other conditions, demonstrated by numerous studies.[61] However, people have different thresholds for the effects of hypnosis, just as there are different thresholds for experiencing pain. Therefore, the use of hypnotic techniques, while worthy of a trial in some more prolonged circumstances at the very least, may not provide adequate longer-term pain control; this would have been of no value to these two patients.

Acupuncture, with more than 3,000 years of Chinese history behind it,[62] offers another avenue for pain control where fine needles are inserted into body locations known as "acupoints," in some way modifying pain by changing the balance between two opposing and inseparable forces, the so-called "yin and yang." For reasons that are not understood, the application of acupuncture techniques seems to help some patients but not others. Many other pain-modifying treatments are in a continuous state of trial for the millions with chronic pain, including musical therapy (listening to songs that bring pleasure), and there is an army of entrepreneurs ready to enrich themselves by selling a myriad of "natural" pain relievers to obviate pharmaceutical medications for those who seek non-traditional measures.

Psychotics and those with variable and acute states of psychosis may experience a complete absence of pain, in spite of horrific injuries, but this is not exactly a useful method of treatment for those without mental instability or religion (although many psychotics "see God" on a regular basis). There is a disastrous and fortunately rare congenital medical condition known as the CIP Syndrome[63] that allows patients to feel virtually no pain whatsoever under any circumstance. Patients with CIP can feel light sensations like touch, and usually can feel temperature variations, but unfortunately, since birth, they are unable to sense any pain. Although this might sound like a good thing, the condition is extremely dangerous and these patients often have unrecognized widespread injuries, fractures, mouth injuries (especially of the tongue), jaw injuries, and they live lives filled with daily damages to their body. However, at the end of their lives (which may come sooner than with most people without CIP because of a lifetime of injuries from painless trauma), they will at least move through their mortality to their death without pain.

It would be challenging for most patients who develop pain from a disease as they enter a state of impending mortality to suddenly become deeply religious in a manner that might modify the pain. Challenging and yet not impossible — many patients with mild religious beliefs suddenly become intensely religious as mortality with pain descends on their life. Certainly, Mr. Blackburn did not have much of an opportunity to even think about it. Mrs. Silverstein did have time, and from her husband's comments after her death, it is likely that there was some potential for relief. And yet while the need for pain relief can become profound under the burden of painful conditions, all these other methodologies may be impractical, unworkable, or a gigantic waste of time and money.

When continuous pain develops, a solution (*in addition to religion if possible)* would be morphine, and many physicians leave the administration protocols of this pain-relieving drug up to the competent services provided by hospice nurses and physicians. One of the cornerstones of the hospice system is to provide pain relief for their patients (who may or may not have religious faith to provide hope for the relief of their pain). And, morphine (a derivative of opium) is the drug of choice.

Opium (a natural juice secreted by the seedpods of poppies) has helped relieve pain since before Byzantine times (referring to the early days of Byzantium, later Constantinople, and finally Istanbul) in a formula that was lost hundreds of years later. In the class of drugs known as "the opiates," the chemical works by binding to specific brain receptor sites, called opioid receptors. When binding occurs, dramatic pain relief occurs, patients become more comfortable, and the progression through the otherwise painful experience of mortality is not so painful.

This opiate drug resurfaced as the source of an isolated yellow-white crystalline compound in December 1804 in Paderborn, Germany, by Friedrich Sertürner,[64] and because its properties included induction of sleep, it was called morphine (after the god of sleep and dreams, Morpheus). He first tested the compound in a few dogs, resulting in their deaths, and after testing smaller doses on himself and some boys, he identified its powerful pain-reducing effect, along with the potential side-effects of psychiatric symptoms, nausea, suppression of cough, prominent constipation, respiratory suppression, and addiction.

Because of its effectiveness in reducing the pain of evolving mortality and approaching death, morphine became the drug of choice for pain control, available in a variety of different forms, some of which have been more recently removed from the market by the FDA (Federal Drug Administration) because of abuse by non-hospice sources. However, when administered in a variety of different routes (intravenously, orally, rectally, injected by syringes or absorbed from skin patches), morphine has been the cornerstone of treatment for severe pain, and for patients with advancing mortality, for chronic pain. When patients self-administered opioids, such as Fentanyl and others, the numbers of patients with addiction, dependence, and overdose became astronomical, with Fentanyl deaths in 2016 up 540% in the past three years.[65] From the reports of the 21 states with the highest quality data for 2016, the steepest rises in these deaths from drug overdoses were in Delaware, Florida, and Maryland.[66]

As a medical doctor, I rarely saw Christian Science believers since they often do not seek medical care and advice, instead relying on prayers and their faith to eliminate disease.[67] I did have one such patient, however, a 67-year-old lady named Claire Demming, who stood out in my practice because of her refusal to have routine care even though she visited me regularly. It was a strange relationship. Claire would keep her appointments, I would bring her into my office, and we would pleasantly sit across from each other as I discussed various ways she could avoid an early intersection with her Maker. She would smile and say, fine, you are probably right, Roger, but I'm going to hold off on (whatever I had recommended) for now. No vaccines, no medications, no studies, complete reliance on the method of healing by faith—it was a mystery to me that she even spent so much time listening to my medical opinions. We never debated her Christian Science faith, but we had a good relationship and she knew I would be there to help her if things went wrong.

Unfortunately for Claire, things did go wrong.

She discounted my recommendation for a colonoscopy, and so when her silently emerging colon cancer blocked her intestines, she relented and allowed for the colonoscopy and the gastroenterologist to biopsy the tumor for confirmation of the diagnosis, while relieving some of the obstruction. She then retreated to her palatial residence and gathered her friends from church. During the next four months, she prayed with them and with her husband as she lost nearly 40 pounds. As I guided her with nutritious drinks that seemed to flow from her mouth straight into the colostomy bag she had allowed a surgeon to attach to her abdomen, she advised her friends that she was suffering from "a really annoying ulcer." The prayers continued, she became weaker and I started making regular house calls as she continued to refuse any kind of medication, telling me that Jesus Christ would take care of her pain, should any pain or distress develop. More time passed, more house calls occurred as I documented her evolving mortality and as she rejected any consideration of hospice nurses.

"They can help keep you out of pain," I told her on one of the house calls as I examined her expanding abdomen.

"Jesus will take care of me just fine, Roger, thank you," she would reply with a sweet smile as her praying friends waited in the next room.

When her husband finally called me one day to advise me that Claire Demming had just passed into the House of her Lord, I made a final house call. Her friends, all smiling and looking quite content, retreated to an adjacent room as I confirmed her death. Standing next to the bed, looking down at her emaciated body lying on the stained mattress, a body ridden with cancer throughout her colon, her liver, and her lungs, it dawned on me that she never had experienced any fear throughout the progression of her cancer all the way up to the point of causing her death, and that there had never been any pain. She was almost like somebody in an awakened psychotic state, there was pretty much *nothing* of any distress of any kind from the malignant disease that ravaged her body.

I observed her motionless body, presuming her soul had left this earth and moved nicely into her House of God, I wondered how many more years of good life she could have enjoyed but for this religion that promises to heal the mortal minds and bodies on this earth.[68]

# CHAPTER 8
## When All the Money in the World is Not Enough

There is no greater contrast in human experience than the division between the primary motivations of life and the harsh realities of death. In life, universal across the planet, it is the essence of existence for us to become obsessed with a desire to gather provisions, to expand our homes, to increase our holdings, and to enlarge our personal wealth. This is not just to "get ahead of the Jones" so much as a fundamental force that involves a compulsion to *get ahead of where we are*, to allow for the pleasures of ownership, the pride of possession, and to seek the power that nearly always accompanies wealth. Whether a leper[69] in India or a homeless person in Detroit, contrasting with a millionaire accelerating down the freeway in his latest V12 Lamborghini, the minute-to-minute obsession is to improve personal wealth and wellbeing.

But, as mortality emerges and life shows a pattern suggesting the end is coming, as the final moments of awareness before death begin to fill our minds, there is a recognition that all the gathering of crumpled dollars or rupees, all the acquisitions of stock ownership and all the expansion of homes inhabited by the fabulously wealthy will soon amount to absolutely nothing at all. If the ownership of treasure is the ultimate test of having wealth and power, then we all must die impoverished and powerless.

This inherent poverty at death, *irrespective of previous wealth*, is the shocking reality of mortality.

This takes us to my house call, to the mansion of Mrs. Von Stratton one Friday afternoon in the early days of my new medical practice. Mrs. Von Stratton's husband had died a few years earlier and she had just joined my small but promising practice, hearing from somebody on her company's board that I actually made house calls. A few weeks after her initial office interview and acceptance as a patient, and before her first scheduled comprehensive physical exam, I received a call that a visit to her home had become necessary. She felt weak, she had told my office staff, her driver had the day off, and could I please be so kind as to check out her problems at her home?

An hour later, my Ford Pinto that had carried me through medical school bounced into her castle-like entrance, and after the electronic gates opened and closed, I drove across the thick bricks of her elegant driveway. Unfortunately, the huge bricks rattled my car just enough for my muffler to break away and fall off the undercarriage, bouncing around on the bricks with a loud clanging noise. As my engine sound abruptly became a *loud* engine noise, I stopped the car and stepped out to see what had happened. My muffler was lying on the driveway about ten feet behind my car, the rusted piece small enough to allow me to wrap a towel around it and quickly stash it into my trunk.  Moving around the car to grab my black bag from the passenger's seat, I caught a glimpse, *just a glimpse*, of somebody watching between the drapes of a huge window near the front door.  By the time I reached the door, opened by a humble and very serious Hispanic maid, my hands were clean, the watching figure was gone, and a gray-haired Mrs. Von Stratton was quietly waiting in the living room, wearing a silk nightgown covered by an elegant bathrobe.

"Dr. Dunham," she said with a pained smile, "so nice of you to help me, I really do just feel terrible."

And so the conversation began and then continued, with a review of her symptoms, followed by an examination on her king size bed, neither of us speaking a word about my beleaguered Pinto, its muffler, or the roaring of its un-muffled engine.  She was kind to me and I was kind to her, she respected my professionalism notwithstanding my broken car sitting in the center of her driveway, and I respected her obvious position in life.

When I found her blood pressure was barely enough for her to remain conscious and I palpated the ominous fullness in her upper abdomen that threatened in my mind a cascade of conditions ending in death, while noting a tachycardia (very fast) heart rate of 127, I requested that we call 911 and get her to the emergency room.

"Is this a *serious* problem?" she asked, the smile gone, a new tone in her voice, her face becoming tight.

"Mrs. Von Stratton," I said quietly, "your blood pressure is low, there's something serious going on in your abdomen, and I don't believe we have the time to put this off. You need to get to the hospital and we need the paramedics to get you there as soon as possible."

"But..."

"This is not a proposal, actually, if you don't mind," I interrupted. "This is an insistence."

"I *have* been getting dizzy...fuzzy up here, you know?" She pointed to her temple.

I looked around the room for her maid. "We are going to run out of time, somebody needs to get your slippers for you. May I call 911 for you now?"

She bolted upright, her face looking frightened. "No!" she said. "I am not going to have some screaming ambulance take me away! No, absolutely not."

"I think the safest..."

"Is there a reason we can't just go in your car, doctor?"

"Actually, the safest..."

"I am ready to go now," she said firmly. "Can *we* go, *now*?"

She stared at me for about five seconds of contemplative silence, and two minutes later as a couple of her house staff helped her outside, she sat in the front seat of my rumbling muffler-less Pinto.

Before I could put it in gear, she turned to me and asked politely, "What kind of car is this?"

I ignored her question and said, "Recline the seat back, please, and could you tell me how to open the gates for us to get to the street?"

With that, we initiated a high-speed departure from her castle, and with all of the enthusiasm of the paramedics I had ridden with during my Los Angeles

County internship days, we made the transition to the emergency room in record time.

A short time after our arrival, she vomited two pints of blood and became unconscious.

Twenty minutes later, with emergency IV's with volume-expanding fluids flowing into both arms and the right femoral vein in her leg, she received general anesthesia and the top-notch surgeon of our community opened her abdomen to clamp bleeders and begin removing the malignant mucinous adenocarcinoma[70] he found growing in her stomach. This was clearly a mortality threat, and in the United States, stomach cancer (often arriving unexpectedly with sudden ominous symptoms) is the seventh most common cause of cancer-death.[71] She survived the enormously challenging surgery and the recovery, an extensive subsequent search for metastatic spread of tumor was remarkably negative, and during the years thereafter, our relationship remained sustained by the bond my first visit had generated. The number of patients coming to my door then increased over the years, helped in part by her telling her friends of the adventure she had in my car and how I had helped save her life.

I had no illusions about why this affluent patient, surrounded by enormous wealth and all the acquisitions she and her late husband could gather, would allow herself to climb into a new doctor's old car, broken muffler and all, for a trip to an uncertain destiny. Although she denied it, I believe she had known, even before she had requested the house call and possibly even before her initial office interview, that dark forces were gathering in her happy and productive life. And, like so many intelligent individuals, as the symptoms had started, she had rationalized them away. She had just put aside the abdominal discomfort and the "fuzziness" in her mind as being another annoyance from a body that had become increasingly annoying with symptoms. With her unimaginable wealth, however, she felt secure. She knew that she could climb into her jet at any time to see the chief surgeon of Massachusetts General Hospital, or any other doctor in the country, and that the greatest medical resources of the free world would be at her disposal.

But when she abruptly sensed the *imminent* arrival of mortality, everything changed. She developed an awareness that all the money in the world could not affect her newly recognized and now-impending hereafter, and so she finally made the call to her new doctor, a physician who could be there on-the-spot, politely asking if he could be so kind as to stop by her home (and, a dark thought, maybe save her life). Finally, with the help of her doctor standing before her, she recognized the approach of an ending where none of her potential contacts could intervene and resolve the rush of her accelerating symptoms.

It is an ironic reality that, in the United States wealth does not show a strictly linear relationship with the quality of healthcare received—that is, the lottery winners and others who have gathered great sums of money or property do not substantially tip the scales of longevity in their favor. Money and wealth does have some effect, however. Certainly at the lower ends of the financial strata in our country, it can be challenging to obtain decent medical services although "safety nets" have been available in the form of county healthcare systems and Medicaid payment systems. Even with these elements, there will be long waits for care in crowded waiting rooms, and often conditions which could accelerate mortality may not be detected or do not receive the preventive attentions to allow an improved longevity.

For the poor in general, then, how much does their deplorable financial status affect survival and mortality? Actually, by some measurements,[72] there is a significant effect. It is just not linear. From death caused by certain cancers and heart disease to infant mortality differences, the gap in life expectancy between the poor and the wealthy is real and is getting worse. When this is linked with racial differences, the gap is even worse: in the past fifteen years, careful government measurements[73] have shown that life expectancy was higher for the most affluent in 1980 than for the most deprived group in 2000. However, like most statistics, this is misleading since it is not just money. In fact, pouring more money into the most beleaguered segments of our society will not remove the effects of murder, nor will it lessen the genetic probabilities for cancer and heart disease, abysmal eating habits and obesity, and life-shortening habits such as cigarettes, drugs, excess alcohol, sexual infectious risks, and a sedentary lifestyle. More money is not the answer and the dream of becoming a lottery winner should not equate with a sudden near-immortality.

This issue of health care for the poor, a topic that has stimulated so much political discussion over so many years, has resulted in many government policies of questionable effects and uncertain results. Throughout our political system, the debate about wealth and entitlements has been deafening and rife with conclusions and proposals that may sound good but often do not solve the root issues that decrease longevity. One shocking example of this is how government insurance provisions have actually increased the numbers of poor who are now covered by Medicaid, while *at the same time*, 55% of doctors refuse to see new Medicaid patients,[74] largely because the level of reimbursement is less than it costs doctors to deliver any kind of care. If these patients cannot be seen in the primary care setting, with their newly obtained "insurance," how do their medical conditions get treated or prevented early, while they are still treatable, before the patient ends up in the emergency room with a life-threatening disaster? Furthermore, and most remarkably, data has shown that for patients with Medicaid and Medicare insurance, even after controlling for age and income, you are more likely to die if you are on government insurance than if you have no insurance at all.[75] The result of all this is that an increased number of indigent patients now with Medicaid find they still cannot enter physicians' office for primary care; in the meantime, everyone else in the middle class sees increased tax bills, increased premiums and the decreasing availability of affordable insurance.

Our country has a huge spectrum of available care, and as I have noted, it is partially but not entirely affected by the available money. But, for those at the very bottom of the financial picture, there are medical consequences for receiving zero care. Ask any physician who has cared for patients who had previously received *no* care about these consequences, or look at the surgical roster, the hospital intensive care population, or the immigrant population filled with cases leading to death from conditions that some early primary care might have prevented. When diseases are diagnosed, they are often far-advanced, and they are often associated with irreversible harm.

I have seen many patients with a "slight tingling of my hand, doctor," leading to a simple carpal tunnel surgical procedure to relieve pressure on the median nerve at the wrist and a full clearing of the symptoms. And, yet when the 57-year-old Vietnamese lady appeared before me with a *severely withered hand* from exactly this same condition that had been a part of her daily life with no care for years, the consequences were terrible and irreversible even after corrective surgery. The patients with angina and an impending heart attack after thirty years of untreated high cholesterol, or the patients with an emerging stroke who had a lifetime of untreated high blood pressure are additional examples. A simple low-cost physical exam with low-cost routine blood studies, would bring low-cost solutions to poor patients, most of whom may be happy to have hospitalization covered, if needed, by Medicaid when that hospitalization might have been prevented.

In Los Angeles, the poorest of the poor often ended up at a small teaching hospital near Los Angeles County USC Medical Center that was only partly functional because of previous earthquake damage, subsequently (in 1979) changed to an outpatient facility. It had been a training facility, and the patients there often suffered from advanced diseases that could have been prevented. One of my patients there during my internship suffered from advanced colon cancer. She was an impoverished lady lying in bed with her daughter sitting at her side and nurses regularly attending to the erosions of cancer eating through her abdominal skin, gradually encroaching on vital organs until her death could mercifully occur. This death, like so many others, could have been prevented by a very small infusion of money—insurance, Medicaid, *anything* five years before for the diagnostic and life-saving colonoscopy, if a primary care physician could have inexpensively provided basic care.

Would it seem reasonable for the government, for our representatives, to recognize the cost-reduction and the saving of lives by simply allowing enough in the Medicaid budget to adequately cover the costs of one good physical exam and blood test per year for everyone?

Turning this debate around, what about the segment of our population who has adequate disposable income? Unfortunately, like wealthy Mrs. Von Stratton, our country's middle-class millennials[76] are inclined to ignore evolving medical realities that can create increased survival risks. While my patient ignored her symptoms that eventually threatened her life, the millennials often ignore the benefit of adequate insurance coverage which would allow improved access to healthcare and earlier diagnoses of serious but treatable conditions like hypertension and high cholesterol.

However, like the squeezing of a balloon, this has resulted in hefty increases in the price of insurance policies, making the purchase of insurance for the middle class much more difficult, as health premiums reached $18,764 for coverage in an average family; for those buying insurance in 2017, the average increase without subsidies was a staggering 25 percent.[77]  An added insult to the middle class is the consequence of a fracturing medical system with the inability of many patients to continue seeing their own doctor with whom they may have had a long relationship, often because insurance plans won't cover their care.

Though the poor have their problems with inadequate access to primary care, and the middle class may have its problem affording increasing premiums and taxes, amazingly, the wealthy also have their own set of problems.  While it is true that many wealthy patients are wealthy because they pay attention to the costs and benefits of everything in their lives, they may be unable to recognize medical factors that could jeopardize the quality of their care.

Mr. James Danstrom is a perfect example of this phenomenon.  Wealthy beyond belief, this 74-year-old man migrated into my medical world after his *attorney* conducted the initial interview in my office, prior to his first visit.  Somehow, I apparently passed inspection because his secretary in Seattle scheduled his complete physical exam on Wednesday of the coming week.  Although my schedule was full that day, the secretary, speaking forcefully, made it clear that he would be back from Japan very briefly and that date would be the only time that would work.  Mr. Danstrom, she added, *expected that he would be seen that day* irrespective of my schedule.  My excellent staff managed to rearrange some of my follow-up patients for another time; he arrived in a spotless Bentley right on time, and two hours later, I began arrangements for him to undergo surgical treatment for an arthritic knee.

His knee was not more arthritic than most knees, but he wanted an artificial implantation he had read about on the Internet. He further informed me that he knew of a Dr. Kingsmill in San Francisco with A+ credentials to do the surgery, the man is "just recommended by everybody who knows anything about orthopedic surgeons." Knowing that particular surgeon's confidential deplorable reputation, a man with a prominent palatial office in the most expensive part of town, but with (I estimated) a C- report card for a shocking lack of surgical skills, I suggested that Mr. Danstrom might consider a local first-rate orthopedic surgeon. This San Francisco physician, I knew from other patients who had taken my advice, could speak reassuringly softly to his patients (with a slightly British accent) before the gentle hustle off to his doctor-owned surgicenter down the street for an often uncertain surgical result.

That suggestion got me nowhere, and one week later, he flew to San Francisco and had the surgery. Two weeks later, I got the dreaded call.

"Roger, I'm back in Santa Barbara," he said, his crusty voice now carrying a trace of fear. "I have a fever and I can't reach Dr. Kingsmill."

"I can try to call him for you..." I began.

"No, I've already tried. He's on the East Coast, on some kind of a lecture circuit. He won't be back for a week."

"Jim, I can probably reach whoever's on-call for him up there," I said, trying to sound reassuring. "There must be somebody on-call while he's gone."

"No, Roger!" he said forcefully. "I tried and there's *nobody* on-call. My knee is red and swollen twice normal size, I think I need to see you!"

And so, I met him in the emergency room; the admitting personnel recognize his name and within five minutes of his arrival, the hospital administrator rushed to confirm that the man was receiving VIP care. He then turned to me and suggested that everything in this case needed to be just perfect—I surmised to myself that my patient had a significant record of sizeable hospital donations. The two men obviously knew each other well, and as they began to share jokes about health care in Russia, I began searching for an infectious disease doc and an orthopedic surgeon who might not be inclined to strangle me for the referral.

Any patient refusing local care and then having complications from distant care is fundamentally exasperating to most doctors; it is a rule in some golden ethics rulebook that doctors who perform surgery are usually responsible for the consequences of the surgery.

Cultures were taken, infections were confirmed, fevers got higher, antibiotics were given, and a very unhappy orthopedic surgeon wrote a remarkably terse note that accelerated Mr. Danstrom to UCLA for joint removal surgery and a very prolonged hospitalization. Six months later, he was able to walk again, but his brush with a near-mortality event seemed to alter some of his confidence in self-referrals to "the best doctors in the world."

The biggest problem for the wealthy patients, however, is not just a tendency to see whoever might be perceived as the best of the best such as a doctor with lavish credentials on the Internet, it is their tendency to not flinch when price tags are associated with procedures that may not be necessary and that would cause most people to cringe in horror. Fortunately, this is not a universal phenomenon with the wealthy, and in fact most of the remarkable patients under my care over the years listened carefully to my recommendations and showed good judgment.

There can be great variability in this population. Two of my patients, with titles of a Lord and a Lady (representing a most respectable English association), were among the most remarkable individuals in my career who followed my guidance. Two additional patients, both professors who had been awarded the Nobel Prize in Stockholm, Sweden (and who had brain power beyond anything I could imagine) tended to follow my recommendations precisely.

Some wealthy patients regularly hustle themselves off to the Cooper Clinic north of Dallas, Texas or to UCLA for their expensive "executive physicals" that routinely generate 20+ pages of report (always using first names and always starting off with "It was such a pleasure to see you in our facility today and I trust that your wife and family…" etc., etc.). These patients were then the same patients who allowed me to do my "standard complete physical" (which takes approximately two hours) and then follow my suggestions. I compared the 20+ page reports with my 3-page report and discovered I had covered all the same bases to keep them healthy. Also, nicely enough, when they left my office, they seemed satisfied with a handshake, or for the ladies a quick hug, and with no letter to follow. Many of them liked my conservative approach against additional testing often recommended by large medical centers in the "executive physical" category, unless absolutely necessary, and several took notice of the fact that I owned none of the surgical clinics that could generate bills in the tens of thousands of dollars for tests that may not have been a good use of their money.

Another contrast was demonstrated when one of my very wealthy patients with a family history of colon cancer declared he wanted a colonoscopy every year, against the advice of the gastroenterologist who thought every 3-5 years would be fine. When he asked my advice, it was evident that he was extremely fearful of developing colon cancer and the colonoscopy helped reassure him that all was okay; I decided the benefit outweighed the financial or physical detriment and agreed that he continue getting the low-risk annual 'scoping's. The gastroenterologist then reassured the man (who was happy to do the procedure every year) and he was better able to enjoy his life of pleasurable good health without having to worry about his colon. At the same time, *another* wealthy patient ignored my advice for regular colonoscopies, and several years later, shortly after he moved to another state, the sad call came with the man crying on the telephone that his new doctor had just identified widespread metastatic colon cancer and that chemotherapy was about to begin.

On two occasions, I observed wealthy patients awakening from the dead. Mr. Rondstedt died one afternoon in his castle-like home, surrounded by about five nursing aides, one of whom called me to announce his sad fate. I had followed the 92-year-old man for several years, and with his more recent decline from the spread of a malignancy he refused to have treated, his end finally arrived.

"Dr. Dunham?" the sweet and soft voice of his chief nurse said over the telephone (all nurses of the very rich speak in sweet and soft voices). "Mr. Ronstedt's final moment has arrived and he has now expired. Could you come out to check on him?"

I had made several house calls on the man in the past, and I arrived at his beautiful multi-level home in the hills about ten minutes later. He was lying in the center of his twin-sized bed, the nurses, all wearing the proper uniforms of the day, stood respectfully in a semi-circle around the bed waiting for the final rites of sorts. His lotion-covered skin looked grayer than I remembered, his eyes were closed, and he wasn't breathing. His hands had been gently placed across his chest, and the only thing missing was the casket that would soon enclose his body. Playing the perfunctory role of a physician investigating the fate of his patient who has clearly gone to the hereafter, I called his name and there was, of course, no response. As the surrounding cadre of nurses watched, I lifted his right arm to take his final blood pressure measurement for the record.

However, at the instant I touched his arm, his eyes suddenly flew open, he took a long shuddering breath, and he abruptly sat upright in his bed!

As the shocked nurses gasped and quickly jumped away from the bed like they had just witnessed a profound miracle, and his equally shocked doctor recoiled back and stared at the sitting figure. And, at that moment, Mr. Rondstedt began to bellow out a song that, for many years, had been his favorite: Maurice Chevalier's "Thank Heaven for Little Girls." His voice carried out through the open French Doors, filling the air of the surrounding hills with his song, the melody was beautiful, the words were perfectly recited and in that packed room, everybody stood spellbound by Mr. Rondstedt's postmortem (and final) performance.

When he finished, he slowly lay back with a happy look on his face. He turned to me and said, "Hello, Roger, glad you decided to stop by!"

I told him quietly that checking him over had seemed like a good idea and I finally did check him over, with the chief nurse standing behind me, saying over and over, "I checked him, doctor, I really did check him, there was no blood pressure! He wasn't breathing, there were no movements!"

I turned to the nurse and smiled. "I know you did, not to worry. He seems to have come back to us for a bit."

The next day, Mr. Rondstedt died peacefully in his little bed, for real, the team of nurses confirmed his passing about twenty times, and he was finally laid to rest with hundreds in our community grieving the loss of this gentle man who loved American veterans and who could not forget the song about little girls.

Mrs. Webber "died" in a similar manner, announced in front of a similar gathering of nurses, confirmed by another house call to her mansion. Before I could move past the initial examination elements, all of us again surrounded by perfectly uniformed nurses, the expired patient suddenly lifted her left arm and began laughing. Her laugh was infectious to the shocked gathering around her bed and everybody found themselves beginning to smile — she clearly had found some kind of humor in *something* and we all found ourselves beginning to feel good as I asked, "Rebecca, we thought you had…you had…. Whatever in the world is so funny?"

She stopped laughing long enough to turn and face me, and while continuing to smile, she said, "Doctor, I just had the damnedest dream!"

"We thought you were asleep," I said. "What were you dreaming?"

"It was so real! I dreamed that I had just overslept and that I had missed my own funeral!"

And, with that, she was happy, she laughed again, she settled back in the bed, and several hours later she peacefully died.

Of course, neither of these patients died twice. However, they do illustrate how a *closely observed* patient (as the rich often are, and usually by multiple observers) who is approaching the end might have deep or profound thoughts become a jolting reality just at the moment they're ready to take the final departure from life. The bright light experienced by many and sought by dying Buddhists, the dreams of sweet little girls, or remarkably, oversleeping and missing a funeral is likely the tip of the iceberg of mental visualizations that are common at the instant of death. Not being something that could ever be easily studied, these final flashes of thought from a dying brain creates some wonder about what final vision or thought each of us might experience at that final moment of existence. It is enough to make one say, "Oh, wow! Oh, wow! Oh, wow!"

Another element of interest to wealthy patients is blood tests for cancer screening. When the expensive blood cancer/genetic tests arrived in the medical arena a few years ago, a sample of blood could (for a price of several thousands of dollars with no insurance reimbursement) provide detailed and interesting cancer cell information. I noted that the patients who went ahead with the tests were only the wealthiest in my practice. None was harmed by the information, as far as I could tell, including one man with widely metastatic cancer; it wasn't clear to me as to why he even had the test. He was found to have no cancer cells but he died of the disease within a couple of weeks after the test; the scientists struggled to determine how that could happen. The very real potential for harm, however, might come to the patient where cancer cells were found but no definable source could ever be identified, an event that never did occur in my practice. If, as it is suspected, many cancers arise daily in us and are routinely eliminated by our immune system, what if a couple of these cells that should be of no concern create alarms in this testing process?

One expensive test that never generated much enthusiasm from my patients was the APOE-e4 gene test, the strongest risk gene for Alzheimer's that could allow the prediction relating to the condition before it arrived.[78] Now, the test is even available on the Web, for about $300-$400, but before sending off a gob of saliva for DNA analysis, some additional thinking is required. A patient possessing this gene mutation only indicates a greater risk of the disease; it does not indicate whether a person will develop Alzheimer's or whether a person even has Alzheimer's. Furthermore, like all tests, there is a percent of "false positives" [79].... To be told that "you are positive for the gene that creates a greater risk of Alzheimer's" would tend to generate the certainty of being on a terrible mortality pathway with a desperate need for a cure or anti-depressant medications over the ensuing years, while waiting around for a terrible disease that might never even develop. Also, the first time such an individual forgot where he or she left a pair of glasses, where in the parking lot the car was parked, or any other mental lapse common to most senior patients, there would be sheer terror that, *it's here, it's here!* Finally, to screen for a condition for which there is no effective treatment or prevention seems like a really very bad idea, even if it was free.

Another trigger for mortality, in the arena of measles vaccination, arises among those who should know better and who often have perfectly adequate means. It has become a disgrace in our country that children who are left unvaccinated by parents who "don't believe in vaccinations" may contract measles[80] (that could have been prevented by a very cheap MMR vaccine) and who then can transmit the disease to infants in society who are too young to be vaccinated. These innocent babies may then be thrown onto an early mortality pathway and die an entirely unnecessary death. This preventable measles phenomenon, expanding mortality risks for the most innocent in our country and fueled by misguided and often well-educated parents in wealthy families, is a national shame. California, the site of the Disneyland source of a huge measles outbreak sickening 147 people,[81] passed a new law, eliminating the "personal exemption" ability of parents to avoid their children's vaccination before starting school,[82] hopefully reducing this outbreak potential in the future.

A remarkable phenomenon I have observed in my practice was the *absence* of wealth in the patient's decision to join my retainer practice,[83] conceived of and offered to my patient population a little more than a decade before my retirement. With my patient population rapidly accelerating beyond 3,000 people, it was becoming increasingly difficult to have enough time per patient to be able to see patients promptly. I decided to decrease my patient population by nearly 90 as an alternative to simply quitting the practice of medicine. With this change, I requested each patient to pay a retainer of $2,000 (either as a single payment or spread out over the year) for medical care with no further charges for anything I did as their physician, including hospital care and house calls. For this change, it was necessary to decide which 10% of my patients would receive an invitation to join this new practice model. I made the decision, early in this process, that I would select patients from my original practice solely on the basis of the quality and duration of our relationship, ignoring any selection factors relating to wealth, degree of illness/health, or age. I therefore invited patients as young as 12 into the practice (with their parents, the child's cost being $500) and as old as 103. I invited patients with severe chronic diseases and with frequent hospitalizations along with patients with excellent health seen once or twice per year. And, most importantly, I invited patients who were just getting along financially alongside patients of considerable wealth.

I expected that the patients of greater wealth, those with patterns of chronic diseases, and the most elderly patients in my practice would be most inclined to join, while the others would decline. $2,000 is a lot of money, now and back in 2002.[84] It was therefore a matter of great surprise that virtually all of those invited joined my new practice irrespective of financial status (and irrespective of age or health). Unlike almost all other medical costs (except for cosmetic surgery) where *somebody else* determines value of a service or procedure and accepts or rejects that value to the benefit or detriment of the patient, in the case of joining a primary care medical practice, the patients themselves made the decision whether or not to join.

In talking with the patients who joined, it was clear for them, as it had been for me, the quality of the relationship was their deciding factor. They also recognized the need for preventive medicine protection from disease, and they appreciated the future absence of any additional charges for anything throughout my wide spectrum of services. From a millionaire living in New York to the elderly woman on social security a couple of miles away, they accepted my invitation for the same reason. Also, I was told, the patients really liked entering a doctor's office and not being asked for an insurance card almost before the first hello is said. These patients, rich and poor, greatly appreciated not receiving any billings throughout the year beyond the annual retainer request. Also, and significantly, from this doctor's standpoint, it was a pleasure to care for patients on all levels of financial status rather than just the wealthy; if the retainer had been significantly higher, it is likely that the practice would have been filled with only wealthy patients and without the pleasure of caring for patients who each became a treasure during my medical career.

But what happens to the extremely wealthy or famous patient? Patients like Prince? Or what about Elvis Presley and Michael Jackson, for example? Most of the public who has followed the sad fate of these two talented individuals are aware of the medical events associated with their deaths *in spite of both men having vast wealth*; both could afford any physician in the country and could pay the medical costs of virtually any available treatment. With all this considered, Elvis Presley died in 1977 at the age of 42 (his autopsy information is reportedly sealed).[85] Michael Jackson was pronounced dead at the age of 50 at the UCLA Medical Center in 2009, and the cause of death was reported[86] to be from the effects of the anesthetic propofol and the sedative lorazepam. However, the county coroner reported that Jackson died from an additional combination of drugs in his body, including midazolam, diazepam, lidocaine, and ephedrine, although the police and district attorney requested the complete toxicology report be kept private.

Beyond their fame, the cases of these two men are interesting because they were both relatively young, and prior to their deaths, they seemed to be not just iconic performers but nearly immortal in the eyes of the public. Neither of them was seen as chronically ill with any specific disease process that might be associated with a high probability of impending death or debility; prior to their rapid evolution of mortality and death, neither man would have been perceived to be on this pathway although anybody closely watching their final performances could have been aware of some impairment.

As famous as they were, near the top of any list of the most recognized performers in the world, both men were continuously under the crushing stress of their performances before millions of people around the world. The result was that both men needed increasing amounts of medication to reduce the human consequences of their work and daily social stresses, medications dispensed in a quantity that could move far beyond any reasonable appropriate medical indication.

With this wealth and with these needs, whom did they choose as doctors (when either man could have had any doctor in the United States)? They both select doctors who end up with destroyed careers, and with both physicians being ordered to surrender their licenses.

Elvis Presley's doctor was George C. Nichipoulos, a graduate of the Vanderbilt School of Medicine in 1959. In his care of Elvis, according to one observer,[87] Dr. Nichipoulos prescribed over 10,000 doses of sedative drugs prior to Elvis' death, and in 1995, his medical license was permanently revoked by the Tennessee Board of Medical Examiners after he was reportedly further being found to have prescribed excessive drugs to numerous other patients. Michael Jackson's doctor, Conrad Murray, was found guilty of manslaughter in 2011 in the death of his most famous patient, his license was revoked in Texas and suspended in California and Nevada,[88] and he was sentenced to four years in prison for having prescribed an overdose of propofol. Because of overcrowding of the prison, he was subsequently released after two years of incarceration.[89]

And so, at the top of the money/fame pyramid of our society, Elvis Presley and Michael Jackson, both talented performers with great wealth, were prematurely dead and their doctors either went to jail or lost their medical licenses. Four people dead or discredited in the middle of an arena of vast wealth and power. Who is at fault and how could this be prevented? Doesn't money buy choice, doesn't *lots* of money bring *lots* of choices, and doesn't fame allow the best of the best physicians to be at your side? For the doctors, doesn't having a famous person as a patient give some incentive to do a really *really* good job, to provide decent care, to do the right thing far beyond the required persona and social behavior necessary in these circumstances?

As it turns out, *all four* individuals are at fault not because they are bad people, but because of the fundamental circumstances of such relationships. The mortality probability is therefore often, surprisingly, adversely affected by vast wealth. The performers, uniformly living a stressful life because of travel, exposure to thousands of screamingly enthusiastic people, and having the burdens of providing the very best possible performance over and over again, are inclined to *demand* (not request) medications and whatever else is needed to calm frayed nerves and to allow rest and sleep. Doctors who face such demands from such famous people become inclined to do *anything* to sustain the relationship—and often these demands come into a relationship within a medical practice of exceedingly small size. The doctors cannot afford to lose the famous patient by resisting the demands for drugs (including propofol, an anesthetic, virtually always used only when oxygen monitoring systems are in place and when breathing machines are available). And, furthermore, these doctors cannot afford to ignore the reality that these drugs are largely addictive, creating an increased tolerance for each drug, and therefore will be required in larger and larger dosages as time goes by and the stress continues (as it always does). Once the standards of the profession are bypassed, then, because of the mandates of the moment in this wealthy environment, it gets easier and easier to ignore limitations and the law, to bypass ever more medical standards, and to ignore the ethics of the medical profession until suddenly, look at that! The patient is dead!!

This obviously has a great deal to do with mortality. If an extremely wealthy patient or an extremely famous patient wants his or her doctor to provide care, the doctor needs to be allowed to provide this care within the framework of established (legal and ethical) rules. If excessive sedatives (including drugs best left in the hands of anesthesiologists) are needed, if illegal drugs are requested by famous patients, if excessive stimulants legal or illegal are needed, the pathway to mortality becomes established and death is often waiting at the end of that road.

The harsh reality of mortality that eventually comes to all of us creates an understanding that may arrive early in life before the end becomes an imminent probability. Looking at great wealth, contrasted with

the aching of poverty, the joining of the two at the
moment of death can be instructive about how we
should be living our lives—how we could be surviving
the time of our own mortality. While life should be an
adventure, maximized to the fullest with the
development of our unique talents, there needs to be an
eye on the level playing field found by everyone at the
moment of death—as noted, we all die without the
enhancements of wealth. Since our individual
mortality is a lifelong reality, at what point along this
road should we begin to divest our material wealth
with the knowledge that "you can't take it with you?"

That brings the cases of four people to this
spotlight, with the question needing to be asked, what
do Mark Zuckerberg (worth $16 billion), Alice Walton
(the only daughter of the Wal-Mart founder and
probably the second richest woman in the world),
Warren Buffett (worth more than $60 billion), and
Ingvar Kamprad (worth $53 billion) all have in
common, beyond their unimaginable wealth? Answer:
besides immense philanthropic activities, they drive
humble cars, each of them, casting aside the flagrant,
high-speed, flashy automotive machines that will
eventually be left behind as each of these people enters
the hereafter. None of them drives a Ford Pinto, but
Zuckerberg drives an Acura TSX, Walton drives a Ford
150, Buffett drives a 2001 Lincoln Town Car, and
Kamprad drives a Volvo 240. All of these cars are good
and they are reliable, they all carry their wealthy
owners to whatever destination is desired, and they
therefore perform the function of an automobile—all
the rest is fluff, and depending on how much you need
to impress or how much speed you might need on our

crowded streets, these people have discovered one of the most important recognitions of life: *it needs to be much more than the accumulation of materials, all of which will end up in the great dustbins of history.*

And perhaps they have learned that the final reality of life is we are all together and there is nothing about fame and wealth that creates immortality or that bypasses the fundamental laws of nature.

# CHAPTER 9
## The Naked Woman, the Candy Man, and the Eyes of the Law

The primary object of a house call is to intersect a patient's pathway of mortality and rapidly alter nature's sequence of events that can lead in the direction of death. It is a simple goal, often amazingly effective. And so, when a patient calls me for help with a declaration of various maladies, (any one of which might prevent the patient from reaching my office), I am often motivated to break away and bring an earlier diagnosis, preventing 911 calls, visits to emergency rooms, or worse.

Sometimes, I am even able to prevent death.

That thought ran through my mind one morning when a call came from a very wealthy and extraordinarily beautiful 36-year-old patient, a Mrs. Sabrina Cartugian, announcing that she had developed a pattern of ever-increasing and frightening neurological symptoms. I recalled the multiple sclerosis patients I had seen from Los Angeles as I gathered my black bag, my stethoscope, and the patient's chart. My medical assistant, Bonnie, jumped into my Corvette with me for the quick drive to a massive home in one of the most affluent areas in our community. The maid answered the door and escorted us down a long hall to the far corner of the mansion.

"Mrs. Cartugian is having a massage in the shiatsu room," she informed us with a proper and formal tone as she tapped on the solid wood door at the end of the hall.

"Come in," a soft and pleasant voice called from behind the door.

The maid stepped back to allow us to enter and then quickly departed the area.

I walked into the room, followed closely by Bonnie, and I immediately discovered that the slender and stunning Mrs. Cartugian was lying stark naked on her back on the massage table. The lights in the room were dimmed and soft music played as a tiny Asian woman in a flowery uniform methodically massaged the calf of her right leg with her hands and fingers. The fragrance of very expensive oil filled the air.

"Hello, Sabrina, your doctor has arrived...." I started to say as my mind raced to recall everything Hippocrates had said regarding medical ethics in the company of seductive females.[90] I glanced back at Bonnie who had followed me into the room, her eyes wide-open with astonishment.

"Ah, yes, Roger, it is so nice of you to come by," Mrs. Cartugian purred. "I just don't know what I'd do without you. My husband isn't home, I'm so stressed with nobody to talk with and I'm trying to get a little relief." She lifted her head slightly and ordered her masseuse to leave the room.

"Hello, Mrs. Cartugian," the voice of Bonnie called out from behind me.

"Oh…" the patient started to say, then hesitated as she pulled a towel around her for an element of partial modesty. "You brought one of your medical assistants," she said, sounding disappointed.

"Yes, Bonnie is very helpful on house calls," I said formally. "She's going to be a Physician Assistant and is applying this year. Now, tell me, what are these symptoms you've been having?"

We reviewed her history and discussed her medical symptoms…a numb spot here, a twitch there, various spasms of her muscles, and I conducted a thorough neurological exam after brightening the room's lights a bit. Bonnie discreetly turned a little knob on the wall and the soft music disappeared. It became clear that Mrs. Cartugian was, from a physical standpoint, probably the healthiest woman I had examined in a long time. Without an advanced degree in psychiatry, however, it seemed evident that she was suffering from some elements of a mild General Anxiety Disorder (called GAD among psychological therapists). Her additional symptoms of muscle aches, lightheadedness, shortness of breath and trembling, together with her increasing insomnia and associated hot flashes pointed convincingly further in that direction. Also, her symptoms seemed to have an association with her current situation that, unfortunately, included an impending divorce initiated by her wealthy husband who was currently out of the state (as had frequently been the case throughout their marriage).

Perhaps I helped save a life that day, as the patient's combined psychiatric symptoms included suggestive verbiage in a seductive setting indicating that she might have at least a little element of transference[91] mixed together with a pattern of exhibitionism that could have escorted her down a pathway of depression and suicide if nobody had talked to her (beyond the maid and the masseuse). Often, people *who have decided to commit suicide* appear inappropriately happy, and often this may be just before the suicidal act is committed. Finally, for any doctor who might ignore the proscriptions of Hippocrates, (relating to transference or seductive behavior), he or she may end up with the *body* of a patient who successfully and surprisingly committed suicide, along with a truckload of civil actions for damages, criminal charges, and disciplinary proceedings by state medical boards.

All that said, at the end of my *strictly professional* house call, Mrs. Cartugian was happy with my evaluation, she was gracious to my medical assistant, and she accepted my reassurance. Bonnie found a tiny vein on her left arm and we gathered a blood sample for estrogen levels and pituitary hormones to exclude early menopause, along with a comprehensive panel and a prescription for a mild relaxing medication. Finally, we provided her with instructions to schedule an appointment with an excellent psychologist and a marriage counselor in the next couple of days.

As Hippocrates had proclaimed and as I had agreed, I remained strictly professional in my evaluation of the suffering and sexy Mrs. Cartugian. It would actually seem quite simple in today's world to stay on the right path as physicians work to keep patients from dying and especially as we work particularly hard to keep from killing them. A doctor really has only one primary rule to follow, a commandment or a mission statement of sorts to do the right thing to sustain a professional standing with patients, with the community, and with the law of the land. This commandment, **_primum non nocere_**,[92] permeates the rules of ethics, the rules of liability, and the rules of criminal behavior under the law. Also, since MDs everywhere are equipped with an armada of medical weapons that can cause patients to die, it is clear that the years of training to become a doctor must be filled with instructions that will help reinforce judgment about when the beneficial effects of using these weapons outweigh the potential detriments. This creates a gigantic gray zone of medical activity starting with acts of omission (which may be the right thing to do in some circumstances), and moving into such activities as prescribing penicillin, writing prescriptions for sedatives, analgesics, or narcotics all the way to using a scalpel or to providing cancer chemotherapy or intravenous morphine to a comatose patient. What does the law say about all these arenas? There are gigabytes of legal attacks available to attorneys who specialize in attacking doctors for presumed malfeasance in these spheres of medical activity, with two rather broad areas of exception: good Samaritans, and End of Life suffering.

Good Samaritans are in good shape with the law; they try to do the right thing without payment, and they are protected everywhere. Unless there is some kind of _egregious_ harmful activity during efforts to provide free medical help to an injured individual, there is almost a zero risk of enduring a lawsuit or charges of criminal activity because of medical efforts.

"Good Samaritan Laws" are, in most states in the country, created to protect individuals, such as doctors and other helpful people, from having to worry about the liability consequences of trying to help somebody who has had an accident or some other misfortune in our dangerous world.

This includes helping people who fall off freeway overpasses.

A couple of years ago, as I was driving along the freeway a man either jumped or fell off an overpass *right next to my car*. Everybody including me screeched to a halt, and I jumped out to see if I could help. During the next five minutes, I tried to protect him from having seizures from his grievous head wound while stabilizing his neck in case there was a spinal cord risk from a fracture. The thought of a malpractice action or liability suit for my activity never entered my mind because of the strong California Good Samaritan laws.[93] After the paramedics took him away to what certainly had to be a dismal fate, there was no concern beyond having witnessed a human being suddenly moving onto an abrupt path of mortality and certain death. As of 2016, virtually all the states in our country have Good Samaritan Laws, although some create a potential for liability if the rescuer is not a medically trained individual or is not certified or trained by the Red Cross and other similar organizations.

On the other side of the "do no harm" spectrum was our city's Dr. Julio Gabriel Diaz,[94] age 67, known to his patients as the Candy Man of Santa Barbara. According to press reports,[95] as various addicts in our city sought addictive drugs to sustain their habits, they went to his office where they received prescriptions for powerful painkillers such as OxyContin and Dilaudid in very large quantities. About 20 of these patients subsequently died of overdoses from excessive doses of these drugs—this would be called "doing harm." After an amazingly prolonged pathway of such egregious prescribing activity, without observable actions from the Medical Board of California (whose website mission statement defines the Board's purpose is "to protect health care of consumers"), he finally, after his arrest, lost his medical license in 2012. He was then prosecuted in 2015. Dr. Diaz was found guilty on 79 counts of writing illegal prescriptions and he was finally sentenced to 27 years in the federal penitentiary.

The Candy Man's activities were clearly illegal and harmful, he was prosecuted, and he will likely pay the price for the remainder of his life. But even though he justified his actions (at one point, saying, "If you don't give them the medications, they are going to go to the street. What is the worst of two evils?"), there is a challenge for doctors everywhere to draw a line with the process of prescribing painkilling drugs that are, *at the same time*, effective and addictive. It is almost always impossible to tell how much a patient wants a narcotic drug because he or she is having pain and how much the patient wants drugs because of addiction. Even the patient may not really know if there is pain or an addictive need; the problem is that pain is *experienced*, it cannot be measured, and with that, a doctor's judgment is often needed to sort out the mess.

It has always been challenging when somebody who apparently has a low threshold for pain (or is it a high need for narcotics?) pleads for powerful analgesics because, "Doctor, I can't stand the pain!"

None of us with private, ethical, and responsible medical practices wants to become the "Candy Man" of our community, creating mortality and death for our citizens. And yet, none of us wants to be indifferent to our patients' pain.

Therefore, for my patient who had lost his left leg in a serious car accident leaving him in chronic pain requiring narcotics, I examined him regularly and I provided him with the narcotic pain meds he requested even though there almost certainly was a degree of addiction. For my lady with chronic painful sciatica, adequate pain medication was provided. My young patient with migraine headaches, my elderly patient with a compression fracture of her vertebra, all of them received narcotic medication during their times of increased pain while I did everything possible to otherwise minimize their pain and need for medication.

Most importantly, they all agreed to my "rules of care" that:

1. No *other* doctor in our community was to ever write narcotic prescriptions, and
2. There will be no duplicate prescriptions provided for any written prescriptions that might have been "eaten by the dog" and other such excuses.

This worked well, (with an additional safeguard that pharmacies filling the prescriptions were able to report to me other similar narcotic prescriptions, from other doctors, dispensed to my patients), and in the meantime, I provided good pain relief for my patients. I did perhaps provide for a dependency habit that had merged into the sphere of severe chronic or recurrent pain but the net result was favorable; it is a certainty that nobody taking these drugs over a period of time would not be, to some extent, addicted. Fortunately, I never needed to discharge a patient from my practice for violating the two rules of narcotic-needing patient responsibility.

Alcohol and nicotine can be, of course, powerfully addictive and stimulators of mortality. The risks created by nicotine are largely a self-induced form of mortality although second-hand smoke's effects are now finally recognized and addressed in most communities. Even the military stopped handing out free cigarettes several years ago, and my previous experiences of regularly smoking cigars in the engine room of my submarine in the 1960's could never be repeated now because of observations from the computer gurus about the effect of cigar/cigarette smoke on delicate circuits. Also, along this path, military doctors appropriately noted the consequences of tobacco smoke on sailor's lung tissue and bodies leading to the rule of today for submarine life: *the smoking lamp is out.*

Alcoholic patients are on a death-trip from the time of the first drink that starts the process of accelerating them down a steep road of mortality to the cliff where they often fall into the hereafter at a relatively tender age. A recent report[96] summarizes some of the medical effects that creates earlier deaths in alcoholic patients, including the depressing list of total body destruction: alcohol-induced car crash, physical injury or violence, alcohol overdoses leading to death, alcohol withdrawal and delirium tremens (occurring in 5% of alcoholics, occasionally fatal), progressive liver damage, pancreatitis, anemia, upper gastrointestinal bleeding, nerve damage, and erectile dysfunction, postoperative complications and infections, bleeding, insufficient heart and lung functions, and problems with wound healing. Underscoring the psychiatric addictive nature of an alcoholic patient who (by genetic, habitual, or upbringing exposures) cannot stop the nearly continuous consumption, even the certainty of dying 10-12 years sooner, or the probability of "erectile dysfunction" often doesn't compel cessation of the habit. Also for male alcoholics, considering the specific detrimental effect on levels of testosterone (the very essence of male identity), it would seem likely to attract *somebody's* attention that the decline of this male hormone and the shrinking size of testicles are almost universal in heavy drinkers.[97]

I tell my patients riding on this mortality accelerator of these medical consequences, I tell them Viagra won't solve their problems that include a decreasing libido, I send them to Betty Ford, I summarize the disastrous consequences of a DUI conviction, I do everything I can to stop the process, usually without success. The occasional exception to all this is the alcoholic patient who agrees to attend AA[98] meetings 3-5 times per week—they often can break the compulsion, *but only so long as they continue the meetings for the rest of their lives.* They then come into my office for routine care, they acknowledge they are *recovering* alcoholics, and some of them have been without a drink for 20-30 years +, all of them still going to the meetings, and none of them intersecting with the law for the DUI disaster that is rampant on the roads of our country.

Jumping to illegal drugs, if the consequences of _legal_ drug addiction aren't enough, all you have to do is look at anybody on any drug from methamphetamine to cocaine to really understand the true meaning of awful. It would seem likely that the Candy Man could write an encyclopedia about illegal drug addiction, if he had ever looked into the consequences of supplying these drugs to the eager addicted population. If there ever was a condition that defined how far a person would go to lie, cheat, and steal (even from their beloved mother) for the purpose of obtaining these drugs, this population defines the very essence of hell itself. The drug addicts can be compellingly earnest, but the dishonesty that is rampant in their ranks would discourage Mother Teresa herself from being able to break the habits that become engrained, often with the first "sampling" of a little "smack, mud, horse, skag, junk, H, or black tar."

To address this nearly impossible issue in the beginning of my practice and the harmful effects on my non-addicted patients who needed my time and energy, I developed a specific protocol to screen the surreptitious drug addicts out of my practice.

James Barner, an 18-year-old athletic man and the son of one of my long-time excellent (and non-drug addicted) patients, arrived on my doorstep one day to join my practice with a history (supplied by his mother during the past couple of years) of illegal drug use. I interviewed him, as I do all my new patients, and apart from a pattern of excessive skateboard injuries and numerous emergency room visits for other traumatic events, he seemed relatively healthy. During our interview, I glanced at his forearms for any evidence of needle marks or the "cocaine popping" nickel scars I had seen on the Jail Ward during my internship—nothing there but a couple of small tattoos.

"I'd be happy to help take care of you, Jim," I finally told him at the end of the interview. "But I do have one rule when there has ever been illicit drug use...."

"Oh, no, doctor," he said with a look of engaging friendliness, waving his hand in a dismissal of the thought. "I'm sure my mother has said something to you. But, you don't need to worry about that, I have stopped all drug use and I will never go back down that road." He looked at the floor then his young blue eyes gazed directly into mine. "I'm never going to use any drugs again, doctor," he said emphatically, "I've been there, but now I'm out, I swear to God."

"Good!" I said. "And so we do have one small rule in that respect...I'm sure this will not be a problem for you. We'll be needing to do drug screens from time to time."

"No problem, doc!"

"Are you sure that will be okay? We will call you at various times throughout the year and you'll need to come in that day. If you don't come in, or if you fail the drug test, I'll have to ask your mother to schedule you to a drug rehab facility but you will no longer be my patient, okay?"

"Of course that's okay!" he said happily, slapping his knee with his happiness. And so, I scheduled his complete physical exam a couple of weeks later.

Is there anybody reading this who cannot predict what happens next?

He passed his physical exam, and we called him a couple of months later for a drug test. He promptly popped through the door, happy and ready for the urine test.

"I'm going to join the Marines!" he announced as he handed me the filled urine sample container.

"Great, Jim, thanks, and let me know how I can help you."

I sent the sample off to the lab. The result: no illicit drugs in the urine, with a side-note about the urine's specific gravity (normal is 1.000 dilute, like water, to 1.030 concentrated). Jim's urine specific gravity was 1.000—*very* dilute, suggesting water, the lab said, and they suggested the sample might, in fact, have not been urine.

We called him for another test six weeks later and I walked into the bathroom with him.

"Need to observe the tinkle, no big deal, okay?" I asked.

He hesitated. "Of course, no problem, doc," he finally answered.

I stood next to the toilet as he pulled out his penis and aimed it at the container. I waited, Jim waited, and we both waited some more. "Jeez, doc," he said, "I must be getting dehydrated, just can't go..." he said.

"We can fix that!" I answered. "I'll have the ladies give you some water and we'll hydrate you on up. It *is* a warm day today." (The outside temperature was about 78 degrees.)

He drank and we waited. He tried again, he strained, he sweated, he grunted out, "Can't go, doc, I just..."

"More water, Jim," I said, handing him another glass of bottled water. "A little more and you'll be fine."

He strained and strained, and finally a small trickle of urine flowed into the container, rising to about ¼ inch above the bottom.

"That's all I can do, doc, probably not enough, I can come back later...."

"Nope, that's fine, Jim, thanks," I said, taking the container and sending it to the lab as he waved goodbye to my office staff and took off on his skateboard.

The urine screen came back positive for benzoylecgonine, the metabolite of cocaine—a chemical known as the "fingerprint metabolite" but which might be a false positive, from a similar molecule if tonic water or Novocain from the dentist has been used in the recent past. I took no action pending the full report, and two days later, the lab sent the follow-up test results, highly positive, for precisely the benzoylecgonine molecule confirmed by gas chromatography-mass spectrometry (GC-MS or "GC-Mass Spec") that only comes from cocaine. This molecule will show up (even in ¼ inch of urine) for 3-5 days after cocaine use, or for as long as a month if the use was heavy.

I braced myself and wrote the good-bye letter. The next day, the mother called, furious that I should accuse her son of even thinking of using cocaine and then to *fire him from the practice, what are you thinking, doctor?*

I explained I was thinking that based on the initial and final lab results, her son was using cocaine and needed help. I don't know if he ever received any help, I don't know if he actually made the effort to join the Marines, and I don't know if he perhaps flunked a Marine urine test for cocaine. All I knew for sure is that a vast amount of time was spent on one patient who was certainly using cocaine, time wasted to the potential detriment of my other patients, and that his mother believed everything her son told her.

Such is the pattern of illicit drug use—an ever-increasing scourge for our country's young people. It has become one of the primary contributors to the skyrocketing death rate from the use of these drugs, rising now to five times more deaths compared with 1999 for Caucasians ages 25 to 34.[99] This is an intersection with the mortality pathway on a grand scale.

The reasons for this are complex but if every parent of every young person in the United States were to discuss, early in childhood, the effects of drug use on mortality and the finality of death, including the high risks of prison time and DUI penalties, and should our seemingly disabled government ever become serious about the failure of the nearly ineffective "war on drugs" (proclaimed by President Nixon in 1971—45 years ago), we might see a reversal of this trend.

Now with James Barner angry, and his mother angry, it was apparent that either of these two angry people might entertain malpractice actions against me, almost as a means to vent their frustrations. I had to ask myself…was I a good doctor, or by this dismissal of a patient for reasons of the addictive behavior and the ongoing blatant dishonesty, was I a doctor who might deserve to be sued for any negative outcomes in young James Barner's life?

And so, looking at the Candy Man's activities or my activities with young Jim, you may ask, if patients are challenged to determine who is a good doctor and who is not, where are the malpractice suits in all this? What about the idea of using the legal system to assess damages, improve care, and weed out the bad doctors, that should work, right? Isn't a suit for malpractice supposed to highlight the bad physicians in the community? While a criminal court may remove a bad doctor from society, what about a malpractice court? If patients are looking for doctors to help prevent disease from creating a ride on the mortality van, why not look at these damages *highlighting misbehaving doctors*, those "bad docs" that may create mortality and death— shouldn't they be avoided? Isn't this what the legal system is supposed to do to help prevent a doctor-initiated mortality? Isn't the concept of *primum non nocere* with a monitoring by *somebody* (like maybe the lawyers, the courts, the settlements), to protect patients from a mortality that should not happen?

The answer is, of course, sure, that sounds great. But it doesn't work that way.

The risk of a doctor being sued, and damages being paid for presumably bad care, should be evident in the malpractice premiums being paid. Bad doctors pay more, right, isn't that how most insurance works? All a patient would have to do to protect himself or herself from bad care would be to look at the history of lawsuits and the premiums any doctor is paying for insurance protection, right?

Again, the logical answer is yes, in reality, the answer is no.

Some of the best and brightest physicians who practice in high-risk specialties are the ones most likely to be attacked in a malpractice issue, compared to those who have low risks because they practice low-risk medicine. The high-risk physicians include any doctor who cares for patients in surgical or medical intensive care units, doctors in complex high-risk specialties such as emergency room care, neurosurgical care, cardiovascular surgery, obstetrics, or doctors in oncology chemotherapy specialties. Malpractice claims against these physicians are not uncommon, even though most of the defendants are outstanding doctors. The result: if a doctor you're looking at to provide excellent care has had several suits, he or she may simply be involved in one of the higher risk professions—it is difficult to differentiate between them with certainty and recommendations from another physician would carry more weight.

If you live in a state where the malpractice premiums are really low, and the malpractice judgments are really low, should that suggest protection has been successful from wayward physicians? As a doctor living in California, (where my annual malpractice premium was below $4,000 per year, and I practiced 40 years without a single lawsuit), there is a cap on the size of settlements for "pain and suffering." However, if I moved to Florida, where the legislation has not placed caps on settlements, my premium would be $50,000-$60,000 per year,[100] and I would probably be sued many times over. If I were a surgeon, I'd pay $14,000 here, and around $200,000 in

Florida. This is bad, but it is even worse if the additional risks and expense of "defensive medicine" are calculated. Defensive medicine is care with many unnecessary studies performed to lower the risks of suits— it currently is estimated the defensive medicine cost in the United States is around $45 billion per year[101] and the harm to patients simply from doctors engaging in defensive medicine is likely significant.

If you were a patient looking for a new doctor, and you wanted to find the best possible physician, would you look for a doctor in California or a doctor in Florida? What about Nevada, where the freeways extending out of Las Vegas are filled with billboards advertising malpractice attorneys who will presumably safeguard your health? What about asking a friend, where outcome of previous care plays a role and bedside manner plays a huge role? The answer to all this is, of course, the rewards attorneys may have by such lawsuits—California and other states have put caps on settlement awards, less money for attorneys (and patients), less enthusiasm to sue, less premiums for doctors to pay. If there ever was an issue about "tort reform" that screams out across the country, this is it—a level playing field with national standards for determining inadequate or improper care would greatly help patients in determining at least some element of the better vs. the not-so-good doctors.

When a doctor opens his or her mail, the only return address that will bring a sudden chill to the body (more than that from seeing the letters IRS) is an envelope with an attorney's return address in the upper left-hand corner. The envelope (often marked "confidential") is usually ripped open with hands that suddenly become sweaty, and a high-speed read of the letter ensues. "No, no, no!" screams through the physician's mind as his or her eyes search for the patient's name, as the words "records requested" pops up, and other words like litigation, probable cause, or damages flies up from the letter to vigorously slap the doctor's face…many times in rapid succession. A quick search of the accusing patient's record is usually accompanied by a pounding heart and shaking hands, all eventually replaced by deep-seated anger (why is she attacking me? I not only didn't *put the worms in her cereal*, I was doing the best I could!) and by frustration that now, *as patients seek to attack me, I am supposed to continue taking care of them*?

And so I was attacked, once, a long time ago, by one very unhappy Mrs. Betty Bartford.

The letter came and records were sent regarding my patient, an overweight 33-year-old woman who had demonstrated finger-stick fasting blood sugars of 135 and 139 — I had been trying to treat her early type II diabetes by weight loss, dietary modifications, and I made considerable efforts to get her to stop smoking. She also had a spectrum of marital problems and I had referred her to counseling. She had stopped coming to my office a few weeks before and so there was never an explanation as to any motivations she might have had to file a lawsuit.

The question kept circling in my mind, why would she sue me?

I had no clue and apparently neither did the attorney to whom the information was sent. More attacks continued with more "send my records" requests to more attorneys…. I think most malpractice attorneys in town saw her records at one time or another and we became quite efficient at sending her special packet to an ever-increasing volume of attorneys.  None would take the case, however, and I thought all of this paperwork was over and that I was out of trouble...until I received a subpoena to appear in Small Claims Court to answer a claim for $5,000 (the upper limit at that time for small claims actions).

I cleared my afternoon schedule, I sat in a jammed courtroom on one side and she sat on the other side, along with nearly 100 other unhappy people.  I waited all afternoon, listening to every small claim of the day in Santa Barbara until finally it was Betty Bartford and me in an empty courtroom, sitting before the judge.

"And what is your claim against this doctor?" the judge asked Mrs. Bartford.

"Mental stress, your honor, he has put me under so much mental stress by telling me that I have diabetes, *which I don't* have!  Here are my billings from my psychologist."

She shoved a stack of pages across the table in front of her, which the judge accepted as evidence.  He then turned to me and said, "Well, doctor, what do you have to say about that?"

"Your honor, her blood sugars were 135 and 139, I was concerned about her early type II diabetes, and so I tried..."

"But I don't have diabetes, your honor!" she interrupted.

"You *don't* have diabetes?" the judge asked her.

She pulled out a sheet of paper.  "I was so worried about his *incorrect* diagnosis that I got a second opinion, from the reputable Stason Clinic, here in Santa Barbara, from Dr. Stanley, an endocrinologist. Any blood sugars below 140 is NOT diabetes, here is his statement in his record! All this stress was for NOTHING, and yet now I have $5,000 in psychiatry bills!"

The judge looked at me, his face passive, and he waited.

"Your honor," I said, mentally thanking God for having learned electronics in the Navy, "with her weight, her family history, and her smoking, I was concerned about these readings and the increased risks of a heart attack or a stroke. The blood glucose testing system she used for those readings measured her capillary reading at 139. This method of testing requires a correction factor because of the negative bias factor from the bridge circuitry in capillary finger-stick measurements and is actually a blood sugar of 143, above the diagnosis threshold for diabetes.[102] Therefore, I tried to get her to diet and stop smoking, and…."

"He sent me to a psychiatrist because of the stress he caused!" she said heatedly

"Your honor, her medical record shows the intense stress from a marital breakup underway led to the psychiatric recommendations…."

The slamming down of the judge's gavel interrupted me. "It is late in the day," he said, sounding exasperated as he glared at Betty Bartford. "139 versus 143, and you're trying to sue the doctor? He tried to get you to stop smoking and to lose weight! I have heard both sides of this argument, I have *personal family experience* that confirms everything the doctor has said is correct, and I am therefor ruling against the plaintiff."

His gavel slammed down again. "And I am ordering this plaintiff to not make any efforts to try and carry this claim forward in any malpractice action from this point forevermore!"

As she stood up and started yelling, I wanted to go hide someplace. The bailiff, a huge muscular man in uniform rushed up and physically slammed her back into her chair as the judge departed the scene. For the next minute, before I could escape the one and only court experience in my 40 years of practice, I had to endure the most hostile human glares I have ever seen—her eyes were ON FIRE....

And all I had done was to try to get her to lose weight and stop smoking, an effort to interrupt her mortality pathway, while trying to preserve her marriage. Fortunately for me in this case, the decision came from the court and not from the patient, reflecting a consensus statement from John Adams, made so long ago, that *we are a government of laws and not of men.*[103]

The challenging day when elderly Mrs. Stanson fell to the ground in the nursing home brings another series of events suggesting enhanced mortality governed by legal mandates that lead to irrational actions. She was suffering from advanced Alzheimer's disease, and there was no family beyond an alcoholic daughter back east, but she had still been able to walk with assistance. Unfortunately, one afternoon, as two aides walked her in the direction of her bed, she suddenly fell to the floor. Being a heavier woman, and with a relatively severe dementia, it was difficult for her to stand again and so I was called, along with the paramedics. Surprisingly, I arrived first and checked her over on the floor—no broken bones, no significant bruises, nothing too worrisome beyond her severe mental impairment.

However, before we could put her into a wheelchair for a return to her bed, we could hear an approaching siren and almost immediately paramedics surrounded us. I stepped back after giving them a summary about her physical and mental status, and five minutes later one of the paramedics announced that they were going to transport the patient to the emergency room for further evaluation.

"Why is that needed?" I asked. "Her advanced directive orders her to be on comfort care mandates and with her accelerating Alzheimer's disease, we're all just trying to keep her comfortable."

"Dr. Dunham, I understand what you're saying. However, this facility has her POLST form[104] and "Box B" Selective Treatment does not have a checkmark.

I think my response at that time was something like, "Box B has no checkmarks?" or something equally clueless. In reality, I had no idea what "Box B" was, although it did cross my mind to ask if it would help if I went ahead and checked the box. I waited for his response to my inquiry.

"No check, doctor, and so we'll be transporting her."

"But…the advanced directive…."

He looked me straight in the eyes. "The advanced directive does not affect what we do, the POLST does. Box B is not checked, we are legally required to transport your Mrs. Stanson to the hospital."

It was hopeless, the law is the law, and for substantial transporting fees, and some discomfort to Mrs. Stanson, they put her on a gurney, they rolled her into the back of the paramedic ambulance, and they transported her to the hospital emergency room. I arrived right behind them, the hospital personnel checked her in, she was put into an examining room, and as I finished looking her over again, the Emergency Room doctor, a friendly gent named Stan Fletcher, popped in.

"Hi, Roger, this your patient?" he said.

"She is, Stan, a witnessed fall, no head injuries or any other injuries, all looks fine except for her cognitive processes which are unchanged."

From across the room, a confused Mrs. Stanson smiled at me, knowing I would take care of everything.

"Great, thanks," Stan said to me. "What do you think we should do with her?"

"Uh… Send her back and…."

"Great, done, thanks, Roger. See you later." He spun around and was gone.

I love emergency room docs—they almost always have a sense of humor (that helps protect them from some of the truly devastating cases they see), they tend to be decisive and infiltrated with a "can-do" attitude, and they don't like to waste time. Back she went in the same paramedic van to the nursing home facility where she was finally put back in her bed. All further movements out of bed for Mrs. Stanson from that day on were in a wheelchair, and she lived another relatively comfortable 10 months before her smile faded and she quietly stopped breathing.

Importantly, her "Box B" was immediately checked upon her return, precisely where it states, **"Request transfer to hospital <u>only</u> if comfort needs cannot be met in the current location"** and, that afternoon, my entire practice's POLST forms came under review for Box B checking activity to fit each patient's appropriate circumstances. A month later, the Medicare system received a bill for several thousands of dollars for the transporting and care of Mrs. Stanson...in reality, it was the price for my not checking the POLST Box B "selective treatment" when it should have been checked.

At that point in time, the only thing I knew about the POLST form was that it was a thick piece of paper with a bright orange color to catch the attention of paramedics answering a 911 call to somebody's residence, that it was usually stuck on the front of a refrigerator, and that it clarified whether CPR (Cardiopulmonary Resuscitation) would or would not be desirable or necessary.

The POLST concept has been confused with Advanced Directives and various "Death with Dignity" forms[105] but they are distinctly different. POLST is a 1-page directive[106] about how people want to live and be cared for in the immediate setting with their emergent serious illness or frailty. The Advanced Healthcare Directive is another legal document that specifies, often over the long term, what actions should be taken if impending mortality arrives and a patient is no longer able to make appropriate decisions for themselves. The POLST form deals with CPR (or not), with Ventilation and Transportation—the famous Box B: "selective treatment" (or not), and with long-term nutritional activities such as feeding tubes (or not). Advanced directives are more complex legal forms and deal with such issues relating primarily to patients who might become permanently unconscious, become unable to make any decisions, or to prepare for an event where a terminal illness develops with a specific shortened time ahead—the advanced directives vary state by state, they continue indefinitely into the future, they will not be honored by medical emergency personnel who (without a POLST) are legally obligated to do everything to stabilize a patient. Since advance directives vary state by state, it is good to look at a state's specific requirements[107] for any decisions about filling out these comprehensive forms; a lawyer's input, although not mandated, would be a very good idea.

Mr. Dominic Silverman was a patient who had no use for forms and legal definitions that addressed the potential complexities of approaching his hereafter. A tough and gruff retired rancher, he had sought his own solutions to his own problems, more recently allowing my work to keep him healthy. He was a tall and lean man, a pack-a-day smoker, and when he arrived in my office, he has lost nearly 60 pounds—his stringy muscles could be seen under his thin skin, his veins bulged over the top of long angular bones. My evaluation showed an advancing anemia from iron deficiency, caused by a slow GI bleeding from the esophageal cancer growing in a metastatic manner into his chest and throughout his liver. His weakness progressed with his anemia and as he continued wasting away, he declined any chemotherapy efforts to shrink the cancer with a sweeping statement, "Hell, Roger, the *beast* is getting me, but my kids are grown,

189

my wife is gone, I've done my life and now I'm okay with the end ahead."

He fell one afternoon, severely bruising his knee and his elbows, and he soon developed some significant internal bleeding from his cancer that prompted me to put him into the hospital. His children, both living in another state, stopped by, we conferenced with their father and all agreed that he should not suffer during the month or so ahead. I told them I would keep the promise, I consulted the compassionate care parameters of our Catholic Hospital, and after Dom (as we all called him) told me not to worry about giving him too much medicine along the path ahead.

"I don't care about that death with dignity crap," he told me gruffly on his second hospital day. "Never been dignified, Doc," he said, "not gonna get dignified when I die...."

There wasn't much pain, his kids went home to the East Coast, we talked some more about life, his departed wife, and finally I started him on a morphine drip, slowly pumped in with a tiny pump at his bedside.

The next day, I stopped by for his examination and he said, "What are you giving me, Doc? Not that it really matters that much."

"A little morphine, just to protect you from any pain you may have. It may make you feel a bit weaker."

"Hell, Doc, I'm just going to lie here anyway, don't have anywhere to go, don't have anything to do, weakness don't matter."

"Good, I'll keep protecting you from any pain."

On the third hospital day, as Mr. Silverman slowly moved down into a coma, his daughter called to ensure he was comfortable and the hospital nurse, Dorothy Sabrina, who had been looking after his comfort needs, stopped me outside his room.

"I know what you're doing, doctor," she said, her voice carrying a trace of accusation.

"What am I doing, Dorothy?" I answered, closing the patient's door behind me.

"You're ending this man's life, doctor, he's not in any pain and you just keep increasing his morphine."

"I'm taking care of this patient, Dorothy. This has been a vigorously active rancher all his life…. I'm not killing him with the morphine, I'm just allowing the cancer to kill him without creating pain.

I had great respect for this particular nurse—she was very bright, extremely conscientious, and hard working divorced mother of a couple of school age kids. She was a very sensitive person who had followed an intense personal agenda of doing the right thing for her patients.

"I know what you're doing," she repeated as she turned and walked away.

I spent the next two hours researching "what I was doing" just to settle my own mind. The bylaws of the medical staff spelled out that giving morphine— even in this Catholic hospital—in these doses was perfectly acceptable. The laws of the State of California were reviewed and again, giving morphine in this dose was acceptable and legal. In fact, there was considerable leeway from both sources that there was no upper limit of morphine in the circumstance of a man dying from cancer. I talked with the hospital's director of nursing who confirmed that what I was doing was fine with her. I knew both of Mr. Silverman's children were happy I was protecting him from suffering and I had answered all their questions about his expected course of final experiences with narcotic medications given intravenously.

That afternoon, I returned to the director of nursing and requested that Dorothy Sabrina be removed from the case. My patient was going to die, I was certain of that, my morphine was legal, ethical, and appropriate, I knew that without any doubt, and having a nurse who was distressed by the process would help nobody. I would not be able to convince Dorothy about the morality, legality, or medical staff bylaws appropriateness of my treatment, and so it would be better for her, and all of us, for there not to be an ongoing stressful situation. She left the case and was assigned other patients. She looked at me unhappily for the next three days as Dominic Silverman dropped deeper into his coma. I stopped all blood tests or any other test that could cause discomfort, I ordered a hospice nurse to visit every few hours, I gave him additional medicine to prevent shaking and to prevent mucus buildup in his throat as his kidneys both shut down and the resultant uremia pushed him further down to his eventual very *very* peaceful death without any sign of visible suffering from a disease that could cause distress almost beyond anything imaginable. His children both thanked me on the conference call early the morning of his death and after I filled out the death certificate, they shipped his body to the East Coast for burial.

The critical elements of this case were that I did protect this patient from the suffering that usually accompanies advancing cancer, and that, most importantly, I never gave him enough morphine to actually kill him absent the cancer. A healthy person could have taken the morphine I provided without much more than sedation and constipation. With the cancer, however, the morphine moved his time of death closer to the moment and it prevented additional weeks or possibly months of struggling from a terrible disease.

And with all of that, I fulfilled the element of the Hippocratic Oath that says, in part, *I will apply, for the benefit of the sick, all measures which are required, avoiding those twin traps of overtreatment and therapeutic nihilism. I will remember that there is art to medicine as well as science, and that warmth, sympathy, and understanding may outweigh the surgeon's knife or the chemist's drug.*

# CHAPTER 10
## The Coining, the Death Dance,
## and the Cultures of the Country

The day Mrs. Jasmine Barnes departed this earth during my medical training brought me a combination of personal fear and an understanding of a population's culture that continued to develop for the remaining decades of my career.

She was an obese Black lady admitted to John Wesley Hospital in Los Angeles, when it was still a training center. She had been suffering from advancing metastatic cancer involving her liver and other organs, and she was far down the long and rocky mortality pathway leading to the end. Working as a medical intern during my first year of residency, and covering another intern's hospital cases that Sunday morning, I did not personally know Mrs. Barnes—my job was to make rounds on about twenty or so patients, most of whom who were similarly dying from cancer, and ensure they were comfortable.

At about 8:45 in the morning, examining patients on one of the larger wards, I discovered that Mrs. Barnes was dead.

Nobody else on the ward seemed to have noticed and I returned to the nursing station where I spoke to the nursing supervisor, a tall older woman with an efficient manner.

"Mrs. Barnes has just expired," I told the nurse. "Is there any family we need to notify?"

"Oh, she finally died?" she asked. "We had just called the family about twenty minutes ago about her," she added as she shuffled papers at the station. "Her nurse had observed a dropping blood pressure, but the patient was still comatose and comfortable, like she's been this past week. Everybody's known she was about to go soon, but you should probably call them again…"

At that instant, the elevator door across the hallway opened and a group of distraught young Black men and women raced out of the elevator and disappeared down the hall in the direction of the patient.

"Oh, Jesus," the nurse said, quickly standing up. "That's her family, they don't know she's dead…."

Approximately three seconds later, the halls were filled with screaming sounds from the area of Mrs. Barnes' bed, accompanied by a loud pounding noise.

"Doc, you better get down there and check it out, maybe calm them down," she said. "All that noise, they're disrupting the other patients."

I quickly walked down the hallway, turned the corner, and was immediately stunned by the site before me. The relatives of Mrs. Barnes had all seemingly gone collectively crazy. Two of the women were on the floor, spinning around in tight circles and screaming,

office and I know he is a second-generation Japanese man, what would I expect that he and his family would experience compared to, for example, a Chinese patient, a European patient, a South Korean patient, or an African-American patient? There would obviously be differences, often-profound differences, which should have a significant effect on management during the approach of mortality and the consoling after death occurs. And if a couple is of mixed races, say a Black man married to a Caucasian woman from Southern California, or maybe a Jewish man married to an Indian woman from South Carolina, what could be expected that would allow the best care possible during the evolution of a severe disease and mortality?

The first step, logically, would be to have a wide-open mind. There are too many variables to predict anything about customs with any semblance of accuracy in each individual case. Mrs. Barnes died of cancer, a slowly evolving process, and yet what if she had died in a car crash or from homicide, what if she had died an abrupt death? Would the grieving be different? Each would create an alternate pathway for the doctor and for the family, and there would have to be huge flexibility to accommodate each variable without preconceptions (which will more often be wrong than right).

Looking at the bereavement process of African Americans (compared with Caucasians), one study[108] found there was a greater support for their grief even though there was a tendency to talk less with others or to seek professional help. Other studies have confirmed the variable nature of Black American's grief from the crying and wailing (with physical manifestations of great emotion),[109] such as the "Death Dance" I had seen with Jasmine Barnes, to a silence and stoic attitude in others of the same race.[110]  There is often a desire to preferentially seek help from the clergy of their church, the so-called Black Church[111] rather than from health care professionals[112] leaving me free to wander away and to not interfere by my presence with their time of grieving.

Mr. Nobu Yamada, my 83-year-old Japanese patient, was a direct contrast to all of this.  Dying of prostate cancer, he was hospitalized for a transient infection requiring intravenous antibiotics, and while he was in the hospital, the behavior of his family was *emblematic* for the culture where a Japanese internalization of grief or sadness is common.  This factor alone may lead to increased risks of depression for the Japanese where there is a fear that even speaking of these emotional symptoms might be considered a kind of mental illness—often considered to be a disgrace to family and friends.  And so, on the second hospital day, his wife and I gathered with the patient in his hospital room to discuss the matters of his health and impending death.

"How is he doing?" Mrs. Yamada asked softly as we sat next to the bed, her husband watching us, his head resting on his pillow, and saying nothing.  She was a tiny woman with a quick smile and a special, often ironic, form of humor—today there was no smile and there was no humor.

"He is improving," I said encouragingly.  "His white blood count is coming down, the antibiotic is working, and he should be able to go home in a day or two.

"Thank you, doctor," she answered formally…no first names with this family. "How is his prostate problem?" she asked.

I paused for a moment, looking for the right words. "Yes," I finally said, softly. "As you know, we did the radionuclide scan yesterday and the problem continues to be serious." A quick sideway glance confirmed Mr. Yamada was listening intently but saying nothing.

"How serious?" she quickly asked.

The news was bad, very bad, and I had been hoping she wouldn't want too many specifics. But I recognized that, for the fear she must have, it would be the fear of the *unknown* that could magnify into the greatest terror relating to mortality and death. If she knew the specifics, the concrete details of this battle, I reasoned, it might be easier for her and for her husband. I pulled out my portable computer and a couple of minutes later, the patient's complete skeleton showed up on the screen, with tiny white brilliant cancer-dots in virtually all of his bones, in his pelvis, his arms and legs, his ribs and spine. I turned the computer around and showed them both.

"The tumor medicine has, perhaps, helped to move everything along more slowly," I said, "but…"

"These are tumors, doctor?" she asked, studying the screen. "Those white spots?"

"Yes, they are and they're causing some of his bone pain. We're…."

"Doctor?" Mr. Yamada interrupted me from his bed. "May I see the scan again, please?"

I turned the portable computer in her direction, displaying his skeleton with its hundreds of invasive cancer white lights. He stared at the screen for about five seconds, then closed his eyes and lowered his head back to the pillow.

"Thank you, doctor," he said softly.

I turned to his wife, spoke some encouraging words, and it was then I noticed the trail of a single tear, slowly moving down the right side of her face. She quickly brushed it away and thanked me as I asked her if she needed anything for sleep or for the stress of it all and she declined. We shook hands, she bowed to me, and I left the room, feeling as if I was becoming enveloped in a painful dark cloud from Mr. Yamada's vicious disease.

He lived another two months at home, I made several more house calls during that time, and he finally very quietly and peacefully slid away. There had been no desire for the services of Hospice, there was no death dance at the moment of his death, and nothing else had been provided beyond the care of a Japanese day nurse and the frequent visits from their daughter.

During all the hours of my visits with him in the hospital and at his home, there were never any discussions about their culture or their religious practices; these were private matters and yet they had a profound effect on their perceptions of death. If they had carried the cultures of Japan into the United States, there would likely have been the effects one of two potential religions on their attitudes: that of the primary organized religion, Buddhism, or that of the ethnic religion, Shinto. Buddhism, we have seen, incorporates the teachings of Buddha, while Shinto (the "Way of the Gods" by ancient Chinese writings) defines ritualistic purity and idealistic paths of existence on earth. For those of the Buddhist faith, during the approach through the evolving mortality process, members of the family and close friends sit with the dying person, enhancing the feeling of peacefulness. Often, a small statue of Buddha may be placed at the head of the bed. There may be an effort to remind the patient of his or her good deeds in life to positively affect the "samsara"[113] in which the dying person's reincarnation moves to a state of freedom from all desires—an enlightenment that promotes the ultimate preferred state of nirvana.[114] In contrast, the Shinto faith emphasizes the natural elements (such as a waterfall, trees, or special rock) rather than focusing on afterlife considerations; the grieving therefore focuses on these physical elements which may be adorned with special ropes or white paper strips signifying their sacred qualities, of great importance to the dying individual.[115]

And how does any Caucasian doctor keep any of this straight, especially when the parents of this patient had migrated from Japan where nearly 400,000 Buddhist monks and numerous sects exist, and when their granddaughter (married to a Christian Caucasian) has diluted beliefs and alternative faiths in their family's evolving culture—demonstrating the reality of culture assimilation and "westernization?"

I have seen physicians carry business cards with a "Jesus fish" symbol (the Ichthys) on their business cards, I have seen doctors pause and pray with their patients, and I have heard doctors try to invoke their own God into discussions about mortality. These efforts of religious-identity with patients have variable results because of the uncertainties and complexities of cultural influences from the migration into the United States throughout our history. For a doctor to even transiently practice a religious rite with patients, trying to merge his or her culture with that of a patient, may interfere with the essence of our country's diverse cultural influences from this immigration. Even a brief review of immigration realities of the United States[116] delivers the message that doctors serve their patients well by practicing medicine while avoiding well-meaning attempts to achieve a cultural-motivated religious identity with patients. Our country is rich with institutions and individuals such as priests, ministers, rabbis who may provide an essential linkage to patients facing mortality.

If there ever was a melting pot of cultural spectrum within a medical setting, Los Angeles County/USC Medical Center would have to top the list.

"Roger, I think you should see this," Dr. Barbara Steinman told me one morning as she motioned for me to follow her to a back room of the hospital. As the pediatric chief medical resident, she had been supervising the doctors-in-training on the pediatric ward of the hospital during my internship at the hospital. The process of exposure to the various ailments suffered by the hospital's pediatric population, many of whom were in families with prominent cultural variations, had already been somewhat shocking, but I was not ready for what I was about to see.

Barbara led me into a small examining room where a tiny Vietnamese baby girl, named Baby

Nguyet, lay on an examining table. She was dead, there was no question.

She had been about six months old when she had died that morning, Barbara told me, and she had suffered from a particularly vicious form of bacterial meningitis known as meningococcal meningitis. Her tiny body was covered with dark purple skin lesions, known as *purpura fulminans*, caused by bleeding under the skin from the effects of bacterial activity. Her mortality and her death had been precipitous but her Vietnamese family had tried to help her through the disease at home as she had developed increasing fevers and lethargy. Not having a physician to contact, they had done everything they could—the baby wouldn't eat, she had slowly stopped crying as she became dehydrated and finally she slipped into a coma with extraordinarily high fevers.

"I wanted you to see the skin on her back," Barbara said, turning the tiny body over.

I stared at skin overlying the baby's back. There was the same purple-dark skin from the bacteria of her disease, but also, spreading out from the center of her spine were dark reddened lines looking like some kind of terrible Christmas tree decoration.

"Good God," I said. "What in the world is that?"

"Coining, Roger," she said quietly. "Or sometimes they call it spooning."

I learned that, in the Vietnamese culture (and in Java, Cambodia, and Laos), when high fevers develop, it is a custom to practice this "coining" or "spooning" activity in an attempt to draw out the fever. This baby's family, following the traditions passed down from centuries before, place warm or hot oil on the skin, and then make repeated deep-pressure strokes with the edge of a worn coin, or with a ceramic Chinese soup spoon, extending out from the center of the back to the side for about 5 or 6 inches. The skin along Baby Nguyet's stroke lines had developed red streaks as this effort to "scrape away the fever" tried to bring comfort by lowering her temperature. Often, older pediatric patients report there is no pain associated with this, as the stroking pattern tends to follow the line of acupuncture meridians on the surface of the skin.

Some of the delay in bringing this critically ill patient to the emergency room, a fateful delay in this case, could be the result of the family not wanting to be accused of "child abuse" in their practice of coining or spooning. The also may have felt they could wait to see if this traditional treatment for fevers might lower her temperature to normal with a hoped-for return to a healthy state. The sad result of this cultural practice, causing delays in receiving immediate antibiotics (which may cure this disastrous form of meningitis), is usually death and a tragedy for the entire family, all because of a long-established cultural practice.

One of the most powerful influences on cultural variability of mortality is the ongoing migration of Hispanics into the United States. And one of the most powerful cultural traditions in the Hispanic population relates to food. None of that was on my mind one Monday afternoon early in my medical career, while I was making rounds on a sweet elderly lady recovering from minor surgery.

"Dr. Dunham to Emergency!" echoed through the halls from the loudspeakers throughout the second floor of the hospital. At first, I thought I could ignore the page, since my office had been working to bring my name, via loudspeaker, to the nurses and doctors of the hospital for recognition purposes of my new practice. But, that message would have been to *call* the emergency room, not "to Emergency;" also my beeper clinging to my belt began to warble—a rare and remarkable event in those pre-cell phone days. And so, I hustled to the emergency room.

"Roger!" the emergency physician called to me. "Can you pick up a new patient—we're gonna need some help with this one...."

"Sure!" I said. And with that I met a 20-year-old Hispanic man named Salvador Limon from Mexico. He was barely conscious, there was blood on the sheets, blood on his face, blood on his hands, and he was writhing around on the bed in obvious agony. I put on some protective gloves as the ER doctor outlined the problem.

"Bleeding from everywhere, no sign of injury. Can't get a history from him. He's delirious, with a fever of 104, BP is dropping. Family in the waiting room, everybody speaks Spanish, some history could be communicated, translator enroute." He filled in the remaining details that Salvador had been brought in by the family, fever for 2 days, no other symptoms except that he started bleeding from everywhere. "He's severely anemic, platelet count is about 5000, white blood count is through the roof at 27,000," he added, more information that was ominous for predicting mortality.

Of all the information, the high fever and the platelet count were the primary harbingers of death in this young and apparently previously healthy man who worked in the agricultural fields with his family, a man who was taking no medication, and had no previous health problem. "Platelets" look like tiny granular-looking structures under the microscope, they flow in everybody's blood stream, and they are critical for clotting; the normal platelet count is above 200,000, bleeding risks begin to increase when their numbers drop (for whatever reason) below 50,000. At 5,000, spontaneous bleeding followed by death is a highly probable outcome.

"Platelet transfusion coming soon?" I asked as I checked his lymph nodes, examined his abdomen and listened to his heart and lungs.

"Infusion will start in about 7 minutes but he may not have that much time left," the ER doctor said. "He's sliding down pretty quick, BP dropping, going into cardiovascular shock."

We pumped fluids into him, we pumped platelets into him, we catheterized his bladder with the urine looking more like blood than urine, we cultured his throat, urine and blood, we studied his blood cells for evidence of malaria, and with the translator, we confirmed that five days ago, the man had been healthy and working in the fields with his family. I put him into isolation intensive care for close cardiovascular monitoring where he received multiple units of platelets and 6 units of blood over the next 18 hours. I gave him medicines to reduce his fever, and I started him on triple intravenous antibiotics to cover strep, staph, E. coli, and every other bacterium I could think of. I hit the books, searching for anything that would explain his life-threatening low platelet count and discovered that, with certain kinds of bacterial sepsis, platelets may become damaged and disappear from the blood stream. At least one thing was becoming clear: his bleeding and his life-threatening low platelet count were both likely caused by his sepsis.

But what was the cause of the infection and sepsis?[117]

I continued pumping in antibiotics and I continued talking with the translator. I finally was able to speak with the patient, who stopped bleeding, and I talked with everybody else in the family (all of whom had basically camped-out in the waiting room). I found that nobody else in their family seemed to be sick, just Salvador. Whatever he had, it apparently wasn't contagious. I confirmed his spectrum of symptoms, including headache, abdominal pain, weakness, muscle pain, joint pain, and he confirmed that he and everybody else in his family had thought he had the flu. *Just a case of la influenze, el medico, no problema* he told me with bloodshot eyes.

Just influenza, until he started bleeding, after which they put him into his father's truck and bounced everybody to the emergency room, hopeful that deportation was not on anybody's agenda.

I confirmed that he had traveled nowhere except to and from Mexico. I watched his fever come down, almost to a normal temperature, and then I watched it go back up to very high levels; I watched it come down again that second night, and then abruptly back up again the next afternoon—following a weird sort of undulating pattern. I gave him more antibiotics and I watched his fever go up and down again. I did antibody tests, looking for very rare kinds of things, all negative.  I mulled everything I had seen in the previous seven years of medical school and residency training, including every Hispanic patient under my care, and I came up with nothing.

He continued to improve, in spite of the continued up and down fever pattern, and he finally was able to sit in a chair and to walk around the room. The family continued their nearly continuous vigil, in the hospital lobby and in the waiting room outside the intensive care unit.

By the third hospital day, two things happened virtually simultaneously.  The word "undulant" sparked a memory buried in the deep recesses of my mind from a UCLA infectious disease lecture years before, and the blood cultures came back as positive for *small, gram-negative, nonmotile, nonspore-forming, rod-shaped, facultative intracellular parasitic (coccobacilli) Melitensis bacteria*. I took the patient out of isolation; I brought his entire family into the room and sat them down around the bed, with the translator standing near the head of the bed.  As everybody listened carefully, I asked three questions that I wished I had asked three days before:

1.  Does Salvador like cheese or milk from the home country?
2.  Does the family have a goat somewhere, here or maybe down in Mexico?
3.  Did *anybody else in the family* recently drink goat milk or eat goat cheese from a family goat?

The answer from everybody to the first two questions was a simultaneous, "Sí, doctor!"  To the third question, they stared at me, thinking.  Finally,

209

with translator help, they made it clear that the tiny sample of goat cheese brought up from Mexico was a family birthday treat for Salvador—a surprise snack for him as he finished his work in the fields.

Salvador Limon was suffering from a rare bacterial sepsis disease from Brucella, causing a condition called Brucellosis, also known as Undulant Fever (as well as Rock fever; Cyprus fever; Gibraltar fever; Malta fever; and Mediterranean fever).[118] Their goat in Mexico had been suffering from Brucella Melitensis, but the family (not knowing this) loved the particularly tasty cheese, the little birthday treat, they could produce from the animal's milk. The same disease in their little goat could have been prevented[119] by a veterinary vaccination, but once the disease starts in the animal, there was no cure (which they confirmed had recently died after looking weakened for several days). The main prevention for humans who might be exposed to the bacteria in the United States[120] is pasteurization, first discussed and implemented by Louis Pasteur in 1864. I made it clear to all of them that this is not a "Mexican disease" and that it has also been found in many other countries in the United States and around the world, although most have eradicated the disease; it has even been more recently detected in elk and bison in the Yellowstone area of the United States.

The latest tiny sample of cheese from the diseased goat had been brought north by a family member who hadn't known the animal was so sick—he gave the cheese to Salvador "as a tasty gift from the Home Country," not knowing of its lethal potential. It was a family tradition: the family goat makes milk, the family recipes define the production of curd essential to

210

the creation of the cheese product, and some or all of the family enjoys a meal (the tiny final cheese product unfortunately and profoundly enriched with Brucella Melitensis bacteria).

Four days later, I discharged Salvador home with close follow-up and extremely strict instructions to continue the oral antibiotics for a prolonged duration to prevent a recurrence (the bacteria may hide inside his cells and then reemerge if the treatment time is too short).

All of this—the wailing on the floor, the quiet grief of the Japanese, the coins on feverish skin, and the food from the little goat back home reflect the cultural identity of the populations within our society, each activity a testimony to the past which relate to suffering and diseases in this country. We are, as a country of highly diversified groups, wanting to cling to our upbringing, to grasp what we hear and see from our mothers and fathers. These traditions give each of us personal identity, a sense of *self*, and probably most important of all, a sense of security. This naturally brings us, of course, security in our lives—and the security extends right up to the abyss as mortality arrives. Certainly, after death has occurred, the departed is not there to observe the actions of our culture-clinging families; the actions, therefore, reflect what each of us would like to have *for ourselves* when our own personal mortality challenges approach. The individual activities are profoundly unique, thousands of them from the language to the food, the mannerisms, the sexual mores, the educational patterns, the religious elements, and of most critical importance, the family's ritual activities as mortality arrives and as death inevitably approaches. These powerful traditions and beliefs cannot be easily moved across families of different cultures—it would make no more sense for a Japanese family to wail and writhe on the floor than it would for coins to create bleeding under the skin of an African American baby with a fatal fever.

The following questions, however, need to be asked: If the mourning process reflects cultural identities specific to certain groups from different locations around the planet, is this identity the result of learned behavior or is it ingrained in that group's genetic code? In other words, do we learn these behavior patterns from observation or are we born with the traits imbedded in our DNA? Finally, is this grieving only experienced by humans or do other animals display similar grief with the loss of a relative or close companion?

A brief review of the compelling work of Carl Safina[121] makes it clear that animals often demonstrate profound patterns of grieving that are similar in many ways to that of humans. One of the most recognized animal demonstrations of grieving is the elephant, described by Dr. Joyce Poole,[122] who studied elephants extensively at the Amboseli National Park in Kenya, as a member of the Amboseli Elephant Research Project - the longest study of elephants in the world. In their reaction to the loss of a loved one, she described the elephant's activities:

*It is their silence that is most unsettling. The only sound is the slow blowing of air out of their trunks as they investigate their dead companion. It's as if even the birds have stopped singing. They cautiously extend their trunks, touching the body gently as if obtaining information. They*

*run their trunk tips along the lower jaw and the tusks and
the teeth — the parts that would have been most familiar in
life and most touched during greetings — the most
individually recognizable parts.*

The director of the Amboseli Elephant Research
Project, Cynthia Moss, described the events following
the death of a "wonderful matriarch" called Big
Tuskless: *She died of natural causes (and) a few days after
that, her family passed through the camp. There are several
dozen elephant jaws on the ground in the camp, but the
family detoured right to hers. They spent some time with it.
They all touched it. And then all moved on, except one. After
the others left, one stayed a long time, stroking Big Tuskless'
jaw with his trunk, fondling it, turning it. He was Butch,
Big Tuskless' seven-year-old son.*

Other animals demonstrate similarly compelling
patterns of behavior during grieving, including
dolphins, chimpanzees, humpback whales, lemurs,
mongooses, and even crows. If the animal kingdom is
filled with grieving processes that mimic (without
training or observation) in remarkable ways to humans,
would it not seem likely that the individual grieving
patterns demonstrated in different human populations
around the world may have a genetic basis? In other
words, the cultures we've reviewed are not as much
*human* cultures so much as cultures that reside firmly
within the animal spectrum, carried to us by evolution
over tens of thousands of years. And so, as we suffer
the loss of a love one, the way we demonstrate our grief
is by fulfilling our inherited patterns that carry back to
even before the evolution of the human race.

This is worth thinking about during the often-
raucous debate in our country about "foreigners and

assimilation," where there is covert and overt pressure for those who migrate into the United States to become identical with those who were born in this country. Since this would not just apply to language, civil and criminal law, or monetary elements of currency, many people in our country would like *everything* to change within these migrating individuals, creating a conformation to existing elements of cultural traditions. However, since our country is 100% *already* a collection of highly variable immigrants (including native American Indians, whose DNA confirms they migrated to North America about 10,000 years ago),[123] it does not make sense that a culturally diverse population of immigrants should try to become identical with such a massively culturally diverse population that is already living in this country—especially demonstrating cultural patterns relating to mortality and death.

It does make sense, however, in terms of our value system and our unique respect of the individual and respect for life, to expect immigrants to accommodate and accept these fundamental elements, which may be considered the *foundation* of American thinking. Other than relating to this critical area, judgments from those of us who are here (either by migration or by birth), need to be put aside as each new element of cultural practice is studied with minds that can accept something that is different. And, most importantly, it is this huge spectrum of cultural *individuality*, especially in the patterns and practices of mortality that makes the population of America truly exceptional in the world.

These cultures may be seen throughout larger cities in our country where an afternoon drive might pass a Chinatown, Little Thailand, Little Armenia, or Little Tokyo—where cultural identities persist. While visits within these tiny communities allow for a sampling of unique food, and the hearing of native languages, it is the romance by the youthful members in each of these clusters that creates the highest potential for assimilation of cultures. The phenomenon of *intermarriage*, while often resisted by parents within the individual cultures, creates the most profound and permanent blending to further the process of Americanization, that great merging of the nearly infinitely variable cultural practices from abroad. And, when the children of these interracial couples then grow, raise families, and become distinct unto themselves, while still retaining some of the most essential family traditions, that is where our country's cultural spectrum guides those of us trying to live our lives in spite of the potential for death. Then, when a family member moves *beyond* the abyss at the end of life, individual cultures, with religions from distant shores, continue to provide personal guidance that may sustain each of us still left on earth and increasingly wondering about our own future mortality.

None of this was in my mind the day that Larry Parker walked into my office for an emergency evaluation with a fever of 104 degrees and complaints of feeling tired and sweaty. Larry was a 44-year-old man on a brief visit from England, with a distinctive British accent and a flare for adventure during his many trips to the beautiful wildlife-filled areas of Tanzania where he served as the president and tour guide for his upscale travel company. He had been in the Santa Barbara area for a few days, preparing for another horseback adventure with his friends in the mountains.

The man was clearly very sick—his face was flushed, he sat before me restlessly shifting around, and he clearly was going to need hospitalization for diagnosis and treatment. And so, the question-answer process of history taking began.

"Larry, we've checked your blood pressure, it's low, and your temperature, 104 degrees…."

"Right, Doc, I know. Started yesterday, it's pretty intense, getting hot and pretty lightheaded." He shifted around some more and I noticed his shirt was becoming drenched from his sweat.

"Okay, when is the last time you were in Africa?"

"Just left, been there for the past three months, had a couple of tour groups out there, travelling the Serengeti, looking at all the…."

I interrupted him. "Larry, please tell me you have a bad cough, tell me it hurts when you pee, that you have pain in your abdomen, tell me *something*."

"Nope, sorry, Doc, nothing."

He was a bright guy, he knew he had malaria and after a quick examination confirming nothing else seemed to be creating his fever, I asked, "Do you take any antimalarial medicine, any preventive meds when you're there?"

"Come-on, Doc, I'm supposed to take Lariam…for months, maybe? Really? And what about the FDA black box warnings, the nightmares, the depression and hallucinations, the paranoia, psychosis and aggression? The people there, the natives, they have immunity. Nobody takes drugs and the mosquitoes are everywhere."

It was a good point, I thought, as I walked him across the street to the hospital. The literature has become filled with psychiatric symptoms from Lariam,[124] symptoms that may persist for years, and the FDA was forced to add a black box warning about these potentials. But what about the people who live in Tanzania, who are surrounded by clouds of mosquitos especially the malaria-carrying species, females with the genus *Anopheles?*[125] Don't they worry about Malaria?

It has long been a custom of the natives to allow *natural immunity*[126] to evolve even though this process threatens the infants and very young children of their communities…. These young patients don't yet have immunity against a disease that ravages their population; about 20% of all African children who die before the age of 5 die of malaria, and a full 90% of all malaria deaths in Africa occur in young children.[127] So, what is it in the older population that creates the immunity that was so reassuring in Larry Parker? The culture of the African community where mosquito-eradication programs have fallen short, where mosquito nets are not used 100% of the time, and where medical centers for early treatment are an impossible distance away has led to the acceptance of a disease potential in spite of its relatively high prevalence in the community. Most of the population have been bit by the *Anopheles* mosquito many, many — possibly hundreds — of times. Yet they don't come down with the disease and they take no medicine.

As the native population of Larry's African community (with immunity) had a culture of not taking anti-malaria medications, he had implicitly joined the culture because of his prolonged stay there (without immunity) and now he had malaria. To the mosquitoes, Larry's bloodstream was like that of a child, the miserably lethal Plasmodium falciparum parasite had started the potentially fatal cascade, infiltrating the liver and spleen, filling red blood cells with the parasite, sickening the patient until, without treatment, incapacitation and death may occur.

I moved him into his hospital bed, I plugged him into intravenous fluids to hydrate him, and since the hospital did not carry the anti-malaria drug Malarone, I conducted an intensive pharmacy search in our community where I finally found a pleasant pharmacist with an adequate supply of the life-saving drug "for our Africa-visiting customers." Larry took the drug, I hydrated him with several liters of intravenous saline, he thanked me and two days later, he checked out of the hospital. The next day he went horseback riding in the mountains with his friends.

Soon thereafter he went back to Tanzania with the unanswered lingering question about his now having possible immunity.

As he joined the Tanzania natives and merged again into the culture of the population, Larry has made it through about ten years since his infection without contracting malaria again. It seems likely that the *Anopheles* creature, filled with the Plasmodia falciparum has penetrated his skin but, like the natives around him, he has remained free of visible disease. Considering this pattern of natives demonstrating acquired (at least partial) immunity, we all have some hope that a vaccination may be developed, especially now that Bill Gates has invested some of his considerable resources (through the Bill and Melinda Gates Foundation) to help develop a vaccination to save the nearly 450,000[128] lives lost each year to the disease.

From the grieving of the Blacks to the coining of Vietnamese, from the acceptance of malaria to the quiet intense grieving of the Japanese, and finally from the humpbacks to the humans, we are an incredibly diverse population that defies easy description. Our love for our family, our pain when mortality arrives *as it must for all of us,* our very essence as humans who think, who feel, who care, and who grieve…all come together for each of us in our unique lives to create the remarkable collective complexity that is the very definition of our culture.

# CHAPTER 11
## Surviving Mortality

Survival in the face of mortality has always been an impossible matter, primarily because these entities are contradistinctive—survival means that death does not occur (at least in the immediate future) while mortality suggests that death is approaching and will arrive in the near future. While it is a fundamental human instinct to survive whatever may threaten us, we all know that death is an eventual certainty and that it will arrive no matter how much we may want to survive; survival is therefore a temporary solution to the life-challenging threats coming our way

This is a big problem—what could be more challenging than fighting against something that is profoundly inevitable?

As a physician, I have the means to slow or stop many diseases that could encroach on the time my patients have left on this earth—I have medications, I can bring surgeons into the arena, I can order specialist's recommendations for radiation, and I have a whole spectrum of skilled therapists ready to help. Some, or perhaps all of these elements may be brought to the bedside of any specific patient with any identifiable medical problem, and yet, is it really the best thing to do?  More to the point, *how much* of these forces that promise potential salvation should be brought to the patient and who makes the final critical decisions?  Finally, who is accountable for the consequences of the decisions about magnitudes of care—is it the patient, the patient's family, the doctor, the priest, is it Buddha or Mohammad, or can it be that one of the greatest certainties surrounding the mortality process is that nobody is really accountable for the final outcomes of an inevitable process?

There are the variables, thousands of them, individually and collectively playing a role in living longer.  But they all come down to each individual's unique circumstances—the quality of the day-to-day life and the perception of the future as determinants of whether it makes any sense to "continue on" with the process of living.  There are many questions to be asked, and as they enter the back of our minds every day, invading our subconscious, they often curse us with the central inquiry each of us must answer: *What are we looking forward to in the future?*

Looking at each day awaiting our entry, we must ask how much family do we have to comfort us, what loved ones do we treasure and what pleasure do they bring, now and in the years ahead?  Is there a pending *achievable* goal in life?  Is there a "Bucket List" that must be addressed, completed, fulfilled?  What about a time of contentment to be enjoyed, a pending task to be done, an acquisition or an accumulation that is possible and yet unfulfilled?

If there is nothing ahead, nothing to complete, nothing to accomplish or experience, the inevitable follow-up question enters our minds with the intensity of the worst question in human experience: *What is the point of living on?* This is not an academic exercise; it is the thinking process that is at the very foundation of life itself. Depending on the answer to this question, and to thousands of additional questions that may invade our private space as the potential for mortality arrives, it has become clear that our bodies will follow our minds as we establish how savagely we might fight to survive our own mortality.

And some people do indeed fight savagely.

This brings us to Bernie Madison, a brilliant inventor living in the Southern California town of Pasadena, destined to become my patient after the paramedics delivered him to our hospital's emergency room. He was a hard-working 47-year-old man, single and prominently overweight, who had been sitting at his kitchen table that morning, gradually becoming aware that he was having trouble breathing. Because of his obesity and generally sedentary lifestyle, exercise had not been a part of his daily program to any meaningful extent. Also, wherever he walked that first day, even down his driveway to gather the morning newspaper, he became increasingly short of breath while, at the same time, developing what he called "jingles in my brain."

He had walked over to his easy chair and thought about his newly arrived symptoms. He took a couple of deep breaths and thought some more. There was no cough and he did not feel feverish. He had no chest pain and so he felt confident that he wasn't having a heart attack. He mulled it over and finally decided that his breathing problem was the result of thick Los Angeles smog. He packed a lunch, slowly walked out to his car and he drove to Santa Barbara where he knew the air would be clear.

Bernie parked at Shoreline Park and sat down on the beach park bench near the Santa Barbara pier to review his symptoms again, taking deep breaths of the cool fresh air. That was the moment when he abruptly became unconscious, fell off the bench onto the grass, and stopped breathing. Fortunately for Bernie, a passerby happened to be a retired medical doctor out on a morning stroll, who rushed up to the man and began CPR as his wife called the paramedics. Within five minutes, a team of paramedics applied their electrical paddles and shocked Bernie, they injected drugs to stimulate his heart, and they finally brought him back into a conscious state. Thirty minutes later, they called me from the Emergency Room; I walked in and found Bernie sitting up and watching television and the surrounding activity with interest. His cardiac monitor, attached to a post at the side of his bed, showed a normal rhythm and his blood pressure was a satisfying 143/72.

"Mr. Madison," I said after we exchanged introductions. "You have had a very difficult morning." *Like, you died, almost,* flashed through my mind.

"Yes, doctor, it has been, shall I say, difficult…a bit unexpected to be here," he answered, his voice hoarse from the paramedic's intubation tube that had recently been withdrawn. "I was just looking to get away from the smog and catch a bit of fresh air."

"You drove here from Pasadena for some fresh air?"

He smiled.  "Well, I *thought* it was the smog down there, Doc.  Just found it harder to breathe.  It was hot and smoggy, and I felt like I couldn't get enough air.  And when I stood up, I got jingles in my brain."

"Jingles?" I asked politely.

"Yeah, you know, jingles."  He waved his index finger around his head.  "Lightheaded, spacy, like I'm dizzy but for no good reason."

"How do you feel now?"

"My ribs hurt like hell...."

I nodded an understanding and glanced at his oxygen level, measured from his left index finger, 92% on three liters of oxygen, adequate but not good. Suddenly, without warning, before either of us could say another word, Bernie Madison abruptly closed his eyes, dropped his head back on the pillow, stopped breathing, and a cascade of blaring alarms began going off.  His cardiac monitor showed his rhythm had abruptly deteriorated to about 10 beats per minute, far below the level of 50 or so needed to maintain blood pressure and a conscious state.

I dropped my notepad, checked his carotid artery, hollered at the top of my lungs "Code Blue!" and five seconds later, I was on top of the man's huge bulk, compressing his oversized chest as a team of nurses, respiratory therapists and emergency room doctors surrounded the table.  In the next twenty seconds, we inserted a large plastic tube through his mouth directly into his lungs while the therapist began pumping 100% oxygen into his lungs ventilated him. As I continued rhythmically pressing down on his chest, I could feel a couple more ribs breaking and at the same time, as my pumping marginally raised his blood pressure, his eyes opened wide as he looked straight at me with fear.

We pumped him full of drugs to hopefully speed up or stabilize his heart. After about three minutes, his rhythm abruptly returned to normal, he woke up and we finally wheeled him up in a gurney to the cardiac intensive care unit. While waiting for the cardiologist to arrive and insert an emergency pacemaker, we were eventually able to get him off his respirator and remove his breathing tube, allowing me to talk with him and gather a detailed history about his past medical experiences. Sitting at the man's bedside, I listened to his recounting a healthy life, except for obesity and virtually no exercise.

"Taking no meds, Doc," he told me, "have no allergies, never been in the hospital, no family back in Pasadena, no history of surgery, and no family history of heart disease."

I finally got around to asking him what he did for a living.

"I am an inventor," he said with considerable pride, his eyes lighting up with a sparkle as he looked at me. "I invent some really cool stuff, do you want to hear about what's coming?"

"We do have some time—the cardiologist will be here in a few minutes," I said, "what are you working on?"

He got just far enough to tell me that I could put an apple, "any apple, any size, Doc," on top of his little scale device and the screen lights up with the number of calories in the apple, the carbohydrate content, the vitamins, the sodium and potassium.... Right at that moment, he abruptly became unconscious again, alarms began blaring again, his oxygen saturation dropped to zero, and his cardiac monitor showed his heart had again deteriorated to an extremely slow rate.

"Code blue! Code blue!" I hollered as the team rushed in again to begin a repeat performance. I could feel the crunching sensation of Bernie's broken ribs, and again as I pumped his chest, his eyes opened wide again and he stared at me, penetrating me, the fear of his evolving mortality radiating into me. A few seconds later, the respiratory therapist had his ventilation tube into his lungs again and delivered 100% oxygen into his system.

"Where's the cardiologist?" I hollered as I continued to compress his chest. A quick glance at his monitor showed an underlying heart rate of about fifteen beats per minute.

"Just pulled up to the ER, be here in about one minute!" one of the nurses hollered as I pumped his chest more vigorously and he continued staring at me. His heart rhythm didn't increase to a normal rhythm in spite of stimulant drugs, I kept pumping again until the emergency room doc arrived and took over the case. After the longest minute I have ever experienced, the cardiologist, Dr. David Quillen, came rushing into the room and five minutes later, a pacemaker wire, inserted through a vein on his left arm, began firing his heart regularly as Bernie Manders woke up and immediately stabilized.

As the breathing tube was removed again, I asked him how he felt.

"My ribs still hurt like hell, Doc, why did you have to break so many?" he asked with a grimace as he moved around in the bed, trying to become comfortable.

"Didn't *want* to break any…just wanted to keep you alive, Bernie," I answered. "You now have a pacemaker that will keep your heart beating at a normal rate. Just rest, now."

He was quiet for a moment and then he turned his head to me and said, softly, "You know at that moment, when you were pumping my heart, when it slowed down so much?"

"That part when you were looking at me, and I was breaking your ribs, yes?"

"I knew what you were doing. I knew what was going on, but I didn't see any bright lights or anything like that. There was just one thing that kept me *really* wanting to fight on, to get back to normal."

"Well, it was your heart, the pacing…"

He held up his hand for silence. "I know it was my heart, Doc. But I also know what is in my brain. I have no family, my parents are gone, and I don't want to travel, but I…." He paused and wiped away a tear. "I have more inventions coming, really cool stuff, Doc, the kind of things nobody else ever thinks about. If I died here, those things would never happen, there would be nothing. Ever."

I looked at him, waiting a few moments for him to continue.

"This heart thing was not going to get me," he said with emotion. "I was not going to let it get me. I have some really good inventions in the pipeline…."

I smiled and said, "I think the pacemaker will help."

He thanked me profusely then asked me to become his doctor, and I informed him that I *already* was his doctor. He told me he would show me his inventions as they came forth in the time ahead. I took care of him for the remainder of his hospital stay, he never had had a heart attack (therefore he had no damaged heart muscle) and his entire problem seemed to be related to a diseased heart rhythm-generating system, resolved by his pacer. His breathing problem seemed to have been caused by some congestive failure from the recurrent persistently slow heart rate, his "jingles" were from his low blood pressure, and with his new perfectly functioning permanent pacemaker, he went home a few days later. For years after that, he would regularly drive to Santa Barbara for follow-up visits and to show me his latest invention with great pleasure.

Bernie Madison lived to invent, he thrived on his inventions, and after his follow-up treadmill testing confirmed a perfectly functioning heart, he began an effective dietary program and an exercise program. "I got more things to invent, Doc," he would say each time he stopped by. He was driven by his future, and with the exercise and dietary guidance, suddenly deemed more relevant after "dying" three times, he became a healthy man. With his cardiologist, I would track his pacer battery life, bringing him a new and better pacemaker every few years, and with the driving forces in his mind to live a long life, *allowing for more inventions*, he trimmed his weight and began to look almost *athletic*.

But, without the powerful force of his creative mind and his plans for each future accomplishment, I believe Bernie Madison would have died prematurely.

The concepts linking mortality with the state of mind opens up a whole Pandora's box of uncertainty. The question that challenges us all is what is the relationship between the human brain (and by association, the human *mind*), and the body? Although a casual overview might not seem that complicated — the brain connects to the body with the spinal cord and by the secretion of hormones from the pituitary gland — the reality is vastly more impossible to grasp or understand.

As a medical student, still in my first year, I walked into the anatomy lab one morning at the UCLA School of Medicine, on Dissect-the-Brain-Day, expecting to unravel some of the mysteries of the human brain. On each of our desks awaited a human brain…our job was to dissect it, to look at its individual anatomical components, to observe the brain cells under the microscope, and to learn something that would make us better doctors. Once I recovered from the shock of seeing so many brains from so many deceased human beings all sitting on our desks in one room, I tried to adapt to the fact that dissection of the brain, as a route to gathering meaningful information, was almost hopeless beyond giving us a general sense of the basic brain lobe structure. Furthermore, the microscopic examination was one of the biggest disappointments of my medical career — there was nothing to see under the microscope but gray brain matter with an occasional cell!

229

Moving to the functioning capability of the brain, I later became impressed by the Internet-led morass of information and misinformation in the divergent realms of study about the brain. On the positive side, several years ago, I attended the $1,000,000 Kavli award ceremony[129] in Oslo, Norway. One of the awardees was experimenting[130] with a little creature, a "roundworm" of about 0.039 inches long (less than one-half a tenth of an inch), called a C. elegans. This creature, almost microscopic in size, provided fundamental neurological research information that was complex, challenging, and fascinating about the central nervous system of this teeny worm and the complex relationship of its sensory nerves to its behavior and survival.

However, comparing this creature's complex nervous system to the human mind requires a mind-boggling transition. Compared to the human brain, the information about how many neurons were actually involved in this intricate and time-consuming study was tiny: the C. elegans creature has a total of 302 neurons. That is 302 nerves, total, controlling all of its physical activity and its complex olfactory (sense of smell) behavior to affect its ability to eat and survive.

In contrast, the human brain contains 86,000,000,000 neurons....[131]

The effect of this complexity on advances in medical science leads to experiments looking at how the brain may structurally change with varying physical activity, and more relevant to this discussion, how the brain—and by extension, the mind—affects the body. There are little glimmers of information, but even the most advanced neurophysiologic centers are

230

mystified by the details of relationships between the brain and the body. For examples of these glimmers, we know that if we exercise, we often feel better (the runner's high, the improved sense of well-being) — somehow the brain is positively affected by exercise. There is a relationship between exercise and relief from the "brain fog" that comes with age,[132] a depressing consideration in its own right, adding the fact that within the brain, the structure known as the hippocampus enlarges, potentially boosting verbal memory and "thinking skills." This observation then yielded the finding that other areas of the brain enlarge with exercise over time — furthermore, stress and anxiety are reduced and mood is improved.

Exercise is good for the brain and for the mind, which seems basic. Good, got it, we all should exercise more for better minds.

This leads to the next question, however, since none of this gets any easier. If activities of the body change the physical structures in the brain, can the brain change the physical health of the body? It is clear from many observations[133] that depression and stress (brain events) may have a serious effect on physical health (body events). Depression may increase the probability of heart disease, depression and obesity are linked, and by such seemingly miniscule events as the initiation of daylight savings time, there seems to be a trigger from the brain to the body (presumably by reduced hours of sleep) causing a spike in strokes.[134] The release of, and the activation of, inflammatory chemicals may play an important role in the evolution of clogging atherosclerosis, inflammatory molecules in the blood stream, and damage to the brain or heart. In another study,[135] the effect of depression as a risk factor for mortality showed it to be even greater than cigarette smoking.

Finally, links between the brain and the body seem to be significant even as related to immunologic events, where autoimmune disorders and inflammatory conditions (including football traumatic brain injury) seem to trigger such abnormalities as schizophrenia (brain consequence) or Alzheimer's disease.[136] With all this considered, would it not be reasonable to consider that the *absence* of depression and hopelessness, in other words, filling the mind with the *presence* of a positive expectancy about the future (as we saw with Mr. Bernie Madison and his inventions) could result in a mortality reduction? Could it be that a profound desire to survive, because of pending accomplishments or any other compelling reason, increases the probability of a continued life even after the most raging mortality scenario?

Such seemed to be the case in the early morning hours of March 8, 2010 in Boston for my 54-year-old patient, Chris Toomey, who developed chest symptoms at 5:30 AM as he dressed in preparation for an early morning meeting with East Coast businessmen. He had been a healthy man in every respect, visiting his home city on a breakaway from his work as the President of a thriving aerospace components manufacturing business in Los Angeles. As pulled on his tie, he felt the slightest twinges of a severe static electricity-like shock feeling moving across his chest. Being an intelligent and savvy man, he mulled the pain for a few moments. It was just an electricity-like feeling, not a "heart attack feeling" across his chest, he thought. Strange...maybe a pinched nerve, maybe some reflux from the filet the night before, or that glass of wine he had enjoyed with the meal. Or maybe something else, but possibly something serious. Although he sensed he might be late for his business meeting, he decided to call a cab and asked the driver to take him to the emergency room of Massachusetts General Hospital (MGH), just five minutes away.

By the time the cab arrived at MGH, Chris needed to be helped from the cab, lifted onto a gurney, and whisked into the "crash room" (cardiac area) of the emergency receiving area. To his great fortune, as his ascending aorta continued to dissect (split apart) upward in the direction of his carotid arteries and coronary (heart) arteries, threatening blood flow to his brain, his heart, and the rest of his body, he was alive upon entry to the hospital. About 20% of patients with his condition are dead on arrival.[137] Furthermore, if untreated, the mortality rate climbs at about 1% per hour, half the patients are dead by the third day and almost 80% are dead by the end of the second week.[138]

If there ever was a horrendous potential mortality issue, this would sit near the top of the list.

The morning of his chest symptoms, Chris Toomey had a total of three things going for him. First, he hustled his way to the emergency room, although the cab driver almost needed a psychiatric consultation after the trip. Second, he immediately came under the care of two of the most preeminent thoracic aortic surgery physicians in the country, Dr. Joren Madsen, who just happened to be on-call to the Emergency Room that day, and cardiologist Dr. Eric Isselbacher. Both men hauled Chris off to surgery in record time after reducing his blood pressure to the lowest possible level to slow the dissection forces. Third, Chris Toomey was *eagerly* enthusiastic about his company's future, his own future, and adventures he anticipated in the coming years of his life—he was not depressed, he was at the top of his game. This powerful force, along with the skill if his surgeons pushed aside mortality, helped him endure the surgery successfully, allowed him to go through the weeks of tortuous intensive care unit recovery, and three months later, to finally fly back to California to jump back into his business.

A perceptive reader might wonder where the personal physician stands with all of this. How does being on the front lines of impending mortality affect the mind and soul of the doctor who cares for his or her patients?

A medical doctor is, first of all and above all, a man or woman of science, requiring a vast amount of time during the training years to gather the details about the human body and the forces of mortality that will eventually try to destroy that body. Including the premedical years of fundamental science, the four years of medical school, the post-graduate internship, the residency, and the super-specialized fellowships, as much as twelve to fifteen years or even more of the doctor's life will be consumed before being turned loose on patients. That is required for the science part, and during the later years of training, for the human element where control of the compassion must be learned. What distinguishes a medical doctor from a pure scientist, or from a random counselor, is the mandatory combination of training and then experience that creates a useful physician. And so, how do we deal with the *human* element of the inevitable mortality process, the part that always involves suffering and often a great deal of anguish, without ourselves becoming adversely affected by this process?

Some of us deal with it satisfactorily, and some of us deal with it very badly…it is often very, very difficult.

There is a wall that must be built in the physician's mind to isolate us from the impact of our patients' suffering. As doctors, we must be objective, but at the same time we cannot be remote, cold, or removed from the compassion that is emblematic of a good physician. The immensity and the finality of the mortality process requires the building of a wall in our minds that shields us from feeling the pain of the human being in front of us, the pain from the patient for whom we are responsible and for whom we must care. This wall, which I call The Shield, allows us to be less affected by the natural human reactions to suffering, as would otherwise be the case.

Every day, as we care for patients experiencing the myriad of the life-threatening and life-ending issues we have seen in this book, we must keep that Shield up, in front of our minds, to protect us from the consequences of being emotionally involved with such suffering. We are still accountable, we are still sensitive, we are ready to accept the consequences of our recommendations, and yet, we are shielded from the pain.

This Shield has other useful functions—blocking out potential feelings of sexual attraction a physician might have toward a seductive patient, for example.

The Shield may be raised or lowered at will, we have control, we MUST have control, but it must never become a barrier to the communication of compassion for the suffering patient or family before us. When I delivered babies, *lots* of babies, during my third year in medical school, I frequently felt tears coming down as I handed the new infant to his mother—my Shield was down, I let the Shield stay down, at least to a significant extent. I let myself feel the emotions of the moment. At the same time, however, the Shield was ready to be slammed back in place if a life-threatening crisis had emerged with the mother or baby requiring the sheer objectivity needed for competent decision-making.

This Shield will not work when caring for close family members, creating a variety of legal and moral restrictions for physicians who might consider being a doctor to a lover or to a parent or child—the Shield will not provide protection, it does not work in this setting. Beyond the minor caring for small matters as a non-physician father, mother, or spouse must do, the Shield will break down, leaving a doctor vulnerable.

Chris Toomey was on the other side of our country when his aorta began to dissect its way up toward his carotid arteries. I was safe. My Shield was not needed.... Bernie Madison, however, *stared directly into my eyes* as I was pounding on his heart, breaking his ribs—the Shield was profoundly in place, to later be gently lowered enough to allow some sensitivity and compassion as he discussed his next invention.

In the control center of my submarine on the Pacific, during my premedical days as a nuclear reactor operator, I knew nothing about shields at 3 AM when Charlie was lost off the deck into the stormy ocean. We had just surfaced because of a bow planes system failure; Chief Petty Officer Charlie had climbed the ladder up to the topside deck with another man to repair the problem. Surrounded by the pounding night ocean, as the two men had dragged their chains attached to their belts along the submarine's railing, like a single railroad track on the deck, the waves violently and continuously slammed against us. Suddenly in the night, a maverick wave, over 70 feet high, came directly at us with a roaring intensity. The men at the top of the sail (like the conning tower of older submarines) spotted the approaching wave and screamed down for the men to get back into the submarine. The two men raced back toward the door at the side of the sail, dragging their chains along the rail as the wave approached. One of them made it in but Charlie was a couple of steps behind and was suddenly immersed in nearly 60 feet of water and rapidly swept aft toward the screws of our vessel, his chain snapping like a string and his body accelerated past the rudder, the screws, and into the black churning sea.

"Man overboard! Man overboard!" the conning officer called down from the sail as I raced around the control center, grabbing the "man overboard" bag. I then stood there by the ladder in the control center, ocean water up to my ankles, trying to figure out what to do with the bag. The wave had flooded into our control center, creating a wave of internal sea water splashing up on the diving station panels as we tried to slow our submarine and to rotate, cross-wise to the huge waves, creating tremendous rolling action that worsened the effect of flooded ocean water on our systems. With the captain and the executive officer on each of our periscopes, looking back into the night for any sign of Charlie's light on his life vest, the waves splashing around inside the control center, the radio voice of the conning officer above us ordering our speed corrections and course changes, I felt that not only was Charlie going to die out there in the huge freezing ocean, thousands of miles from land, but also that *there was nothing I could do about it.*

After five minutes of working to turn our submarine around, our captain caught a glimpse, just a flash, of Charlie's light in the distance as he crested on the top of a wave far behind us. He marked the bearing, and after twenty minutes of intense effort, Charlie was recovered alive and lowered headfirst down the hatch into our submarine, almost expired from hypothermia and exposure to the pounding cold ocean. Barely conscious, the veteran chief petty officer was crying and saying that he had never seen our submarine coming for him, while at the same time, I was crying out of relief at his salvation but also because of the frustration that there was nothing I did or could have done to save him. If he had been lost, I would have still been standing there with the Man Overboard Bag in my hands, waiting for nothing. Our doc (a hospital corpsman) wrapped Charlie in blankets, he was given a beverage that we never see at sea, and we dove back to a respectable 500 feet where the rest of the night was calm. Two days later, we finally surfaced again in a calm sea and fixed our bow planes mechanical problem.

From that day on, almost as a powerful fuel for my decision to become a physician, I committed myself to never again face a human being's approaching mortality without being able to affect it, perhaps to control it, for the best possible outcome. I also learned to create the Shield that protected me from the trauma of regular visits to the profound arena of impending mortality.

These lessons and this Shield then protected me the day, near the end of my medical career, when my 78-year-old patient, Sam Bronson was brought into the emergency room with a fulminant abdominal bleeding aorta. Sam was a wealthy man, he owned a huge aviation parts company in Southern California and he suffered from a number of other medical problems that had prevented us from earlier elective surgery for his aneurism. The Montecito Fire Chief had called me from his residence after his wife's 911 call, after he had suddenly doubled over in pain that morning from the bleeding into his abdomen. After the hospital's emergency ultrasound study demonstrated his huge aorta bleeding into his lower abdomen, we called the surgeon for an emergency evaluation and surgery.

Unfortunately, the fastest the surgeon could make it was "in ten minutes," travelling in from another hospital, and no other surgeons were available.

We rushed him into an elevator that could take us up to the surgical suites, and as the elevator door began to close upon us, with the nurse standing at the front of Sam's gurney and his electrocardiographic monitor on the mattress between his legs, I suddenly had a terrible déjà vu sensation, from my training days at Huntington Memorial hospital. It came into my mind with a flash, the time when I had climbed into the elevator with Joseph Tomascas, the man who was bleeding and dying from his rupturing abdominal aneurysm.

And, to make matters worse, as the elevator door closed, Sam lifted his head up from the gurney mattress and looked directly at me. "Don't let me die!" he said weakly, as my Shield raised higher, suppressing the flashing of chills that started going down my back. "Don't let me die!" he pleaded again as the elevator ascended and the nurse and I struggled to reassure him.

His blood pressure dropped during the elevator ride, the surgeon didn't arrive for another five minutes, just enough time for the radiologist, the nurse, and me to sterilize his abdomen with antiseptic solutions, for the anesthesiologist to render him unconscious, and for the *radiologist* to grab the scalpel and make the first abdominal incision as I patted the sides of the emerging surgical wound. The surgeon rushed in a couple of minutes later, I rushed out immediately thereafter and I went to the waiting room to discuss the challenges and current status in the most compassionate possible manner with his frightened wife.

"His age and other medical problems stack up the odds against him," I told her. "But the surgeon is outstanding and Sam does have a chance to make it through this."

"I understand," she told me. "But we really can't lose him now…he has so much ahead of him. His company, it's thriving, he's down there every day, he has so many plans, he is looking forward...."

I held her hand, offering my sympathy for the threats to her husband's life that morning, and we waited together for the surgical suite doors to open and for the surgeon's report.

And that seemed to have made the difference as the nurse wheeled Sam Bronson out of surgery nearly three hours later with a brand new Dacron abdominal aorta. The exhausted surgeon gave us his favorable report as our patient was moved into the intensive care unit where he struggled for the next two weeks before making a full recovery from his time of near-mortality, moving on to expand his company keeping airliners flying around our country.

The inventor, the CEO, and the airline parts company owner all survived the extreme challenges in their individual battles against the powerful forces of nature. And so they move on with their lives, surviving mortality (for now) and living each day with hope for the next, as the rest of us continue with our lives. From the religions to the wealth, the family around us to the doctor at our bedside, we should not be fearful for the moment we might take our final breath, think our final thought, and feel our final emotion. These are all part of life, and if we have listened to the stories allowing an assembly of weapons available against a life that does not end well, we may have the certainty that surviving mortality—even if it includes a trip to the hereafter— will bring us great fulfillment during our time left on this earth.

And that is all we may ask.

# Acknowledgements

Without the encouragement of my family and friends, this book would not have been possible. I am forever appreciative for this this great help. I appreciate the time and advice provided by Rabbi Stephen E. Cohen on specific matters relating to mortality. Also, the editing expertise of Laura Long was vital to the successful development of the book and is greatly appreciated.

To protect the privacy of the actual individuals and families in this book, names and identifying characteristics have been altered; however, the stories of their lives, their battles, their circumstances, and their fates are all real. These patients have been my teachers over the years, and I have learned the lessons of their experiences, many of which I have passed on to the new physicians who follow in my pathway as my career finally completes forty years of work as a medical doctor. The decisions made with these people were difficult, they regularly involved efforts to sustain life and to improve circumstances leading towards death; the consequences of this process were profound and often permanent, touching on some of the most sacred elements within the Temple of Medicine.

I am greatly in debt to these good patients for bringing me their challenges and for allowing me to help with their care — they have made my life profoundly fulfilling.

*This book is dedicated to my loving wife, Keiko,
for her inspiration, her devotion, and her support, without which SURVIVING MORTALITY would not have been possible*

# ENDNOTES

[1] Described nowhere in the Koran. This "72 virgin" term probably arose from a description of paradise from Imam at-Tirmidhi in the 9th Century

[2] All names in this book are changed to protect the privacy of these individuals and their families.

[3] *The complexities of Physician Supply and Demand: Projections from 2013-2025* from the economic modeling and forecasting firm IHS Inc., at the request of the AAMC.

[4] https://www.cdc.gov/nchs/products/databriefs/db293.htm

[5] Edward A. Murphy, Jr. was one of the engineers on the rocket-sled experiments that were performed by the U.S. Air Force in 1949 to test human acceleration tolerances. One experiment involved a set of 16 accelerometers mounted to different parts of the subject's body. There were two ways each sensor could be glued to its mount, and somebody had methodically installed all 16 the wrong way around. Murphy then made the original form of his pronouncement, which the test subject (the late Major John Paul Stapp) quoted at a news conference a few days later. The basic Murphy's Law says, "Anything that can go wrong, will." However, the correct, original Murphy's Law reads: "If there are two or more ways to do something, and one of those ways can result in a catastrophe, then someone will do it that way."

Within months `Murphy's Law' had spread throughout various technical cultures connected to aerospace engineering and from there to almost everywhere in life. Following an evolutionary pathway of human adjustments, the variants moved further into the popular imagination, changing as they went. Medicine is now filled with some of the most imaginative, and most often reoccurring variants of this law.

[6] Spy Sub: A Top Secret Mission to the Bottom of the Pacific, http://rogercdunham.com

[7] https://www.statista.com/statistics/274513/life-expectancy-in-north-america/

[8] IRS distribution worksheet:

https://www.irs.gov/pub/irs-tege/uniform_rmd_wksht.pdf

[9] Reported by Bernard Lagan, ©THE TIMES, London, 2015

[10] http://kff.org/other/state-indicator/life-expectancy-by-re/

[11] Dan Zenka Senior Vice President, Prostate Cancer Foundation, October 05, 2012

[12] Per 100,000 men, National Cancer Institute

[13] Per 100,000 women. Epidemiology of Breast Cancer in Japan and the US JMAJ 52(1): 39–44, 2009 Kumiko SAIKA, Tomotaka SOBUE. Japanese women in the United States have a breast cancer risk that approximates that of Caucasian women.

[14] Avik Roy, Forbes staff, NOV 23, 2011 The Myth of Americans' Poor Life Expectancy

[15] A powerful opioid, about 100x more potent than morphine, and 50x more potent than pharmaceutical pure heroin, according to the CDC

[16] The risk of pancreatic cancer is doubled in smokers.

[17]Named after Allen Whipple, MD, a Columbia University surgeon who was the first American to perform the operation in 1935, a procedure that removes a large portion of the pancreas, the gall bladder, a part of the stomach, and duodenum. It is seen as a heroic attempt to save the life of a patient with pancreatic cancer, and it sometimes is successful if the malignancy is contained within the removed tissue

[18] Centers for Medicare Services: https://www.medicare.gov/Pubs/pdf/02154.pdf

[19] Audrey Wuerl: Choosing Between Hospice Care and Palliative Care: An In-depth Look at Your Options, from Caring.com: https://www.caring.com/articles/hospital-based-palliative-care-vs-hospice-care-at-home

[20] From his sister, Mona Simpson, at his eulogy in 2011

[21] Fortunately, today's electronics records allow the instantaneous transmission of this kind of information.

[22] Guthmann, Edward (October 30, 2005). "Lethal Beauty". San Francisco Chronicle. Retrieved October 12, 2015.

[23]Department of Public Health, Oregon: https://public.health.oregon.gov/ProviderPartnerResour

ces/EvaluationResearch/DeathwithDignityAct/Document
s/year16.pdf

[24] Dr. Elisabeth Kubler-Ross, ON DEATH AND DYING:
WHAT THE DYING HAVE TO TEACH DOCTORS, NURSES,
CLERGY AND THEIR OWN FAMILIES AND THE FIVE
STAGES OF GRIEF, Published 1969, Scribner, a division of
Simon and Schuster

[25] Mediumship: is the practice of certain people—called
mediums—to reportedly mediate communication
between spirits of the deceased and living human beings.

[26] Allan Kellehear, PhD, is Professor of Community
Health, School of Health and Education, Middlesex
University. He was formerly Professor of Palliative Care
at LaTrobe University in Australia (1998 – 2006),
Professor of Sociology at the University of Bath in
England (2006 – 2011), and Professor in the Department
of Community Health & Epidemiology at Dalhousie
University in Nova Scotia, Canada (2011-2013).

[27] Testing such items as subtracting serial 7's, spelling
"world" backwards, orientation to time and place,
drawing intercepting pentagons, and so on

[28] A dementia caused by emotional distress or by severe
depression, resolved when the underlying triggering
event is resolved or the depression is treated

[29] A condition formally called Bovine spongiform
encephalopathy (BSE), a fatal neurodegenerative
disease creating a spongy degeneration in
the brains and spinal cords of cows in England. More
than 180,000 cattle were infected during that time and
4.4 million needed to be slaughtered during a
widespread eradication program.

[30] A small protein-like infectious disease-causing agent
that is believed to be the smallest infectious particle. A
prion is not bacterial, fungal, or viral and contains no
genetic material.

[31] Cures hepatitis C in about 90% of the cases at the cost
of $84,000 (approximately $1,000 per pill).

[32] Now, the placement of an aortic valve, inserted
through veins, would have changed his entire prognosis.

[33] Elderly people often don't get fevers even when
they're infected.  For a 90-year-old woman to have a
fever, she is likely to be either stronger than she looks or
she is severely infected.

[34] Viperfish is a pseudonym, the submarine's identity concealed to protect the secrecy of Pacific Ocean espionage activities during the Cold War, from SPY SUB (http://rogercdunham.com)

[35] The United States Submarine Service is all-volunteer; anybody who becomes a "Non-Vol" (an extremely rare event), is transferred to surface ships for the remainder of his time of duty.

[36] Harold Luft, Ph.D., of the University of California at San Francisco

[37] Christopher Weaver, Anna Wilde Mathews, and Tom Mcginty, Wall Street Journal, December 25, 2015, "New Risks at Rural Hospitals."

[38] Colin Begg, Ph.D., 1998

[39] mrem refers to millirem, or one thousandth of a rem (Roentgen Equivalent Mammal), a measurement of biological damage to human tissue by gamma, neutron, and other sources of radiation. One rem carries with it a 0.055% chance of eventually developing cancer, according to the International Commission on Radiological Protection (Annals of the ICRP, ICRP publication 103 37 (2-4), ISBN 978-0-7020-3048-2)

[40] Reuters Health, May 18, 2001

[41] https://www.health.govt.nz/system/files/documents/pages/ctscreening-wholebodyandtargeted.pdf

[42] Wall and Hart, British Journal of Radiology, May 1997, Vol. 70, pp. 437-439; and Shrimpton et al

[43] LA Times, Roger C. Dunham, May 13, 2010

[44] The TB skin test is often negative when a patient is suffering from overwhelming disease.

[45] A palm-shaped item of jewelry depicting an open right hand, often worn by men and women as a sign of defense from the "evil eye" (causing illness, unluckiness, or death) and presumed to protect from evil forces in general, with other meanings relating to good luck, fertility, and warding off threats to life in Jewish, Islamic, and Buddhist religious teachings.

[46] Muslim missionaries or teachers

[47] CARA (Center for Applied Research in the Apostolate) 2014 report, 2300 Wisconsin Ave, NW Suite 400 Washington, DC 20007

[48] Merriam-Webster

[49] As compared to "venial" or innocuous sin, a mortal sin

is any action considered to be a grave violation of God's law, such as idolatry (worship of idols), murder, or adultery

[50] Taken from A Guide to Jewish Religious Practice, by Isaac Klein, The Jewish Theological Seminary of America, New York, 1979

[51] Hamadrikh, The Rabbi's Guide, A Manual of Jewish Religious Rituals, Ceremonies and Customs, by Hyman E. Goldin (revised edition)

[52] Ibid. #47

[53] The "dust to dust" concept from the English burial service derived from the Biblical text, Genesis 3:19 (King James Version): *"In the sweat of thy face shalt thou eat bread, till thou return unto the ground; for out of it was thou taken: for dust thou art, and unto dust shalt thou return."*

[54] Tracey R. Rich, Olam Ha-Ba: The Afterlife, Biblical References, Resurrection and Reincarnation World to Come, http://www.jewfaq.org/olamhaba.htm

[55] From Judaism 101; Kolatch, Alfred J. The Jewish Book of Why/The Second Jewish Book of Why. NY: Jonathan David Publishers, 1989, https://www.jewishvirtuallibrary.org/jsource/Judaism/death.html

[56] Perhaps as a cow, or as any other form of life—this is a fundamental concept of Hinduism.

[57] https://www.nlm.nih.gov/medlineplus/magazine/issues/fall07/articles/fall07pg20.html

[58] American Hospice Foundation (www.americanhospice.org).

[59] Ashura is a commemoration of the killing of Imam Hussein, the grandson of the prophet Muhammad in about 680 CE (the term "CE" or "C.E." is beginning to replace the previous "AD"—anno Domini, Latin for "in the year of the Lord" after new information regarding the date of Christ's birth).  This commemoration expresses regret at being unable to save the true heir of Muhammad's legacy.

[60] These rituals are generally performed in countries with large populations of Shia, including India, Lebanon, Pakistan, Iran, Iraq, and Bahrain

[61] Int J Clin Exp Hypn. Author manuscript; available in PMC 2009 Sep 25, published in final edited form as: Int J

Clin Exp Hypn. 2007 Jul; 55(3): 275–287, from NCBI
(National Center for Biotechnical Information) at:
http://www.ncbi.nlm.nih.gov/pmc/articles/
PMC2752362/
[62]Oxford University Press, Online ISSN 2058-5357 - Print
ISSN 2058-5349 Copyright © 2016 the British Journal of
Anaesthesia,
http://ceaccp.oxfordjournals.org/content/7/4/135.full
[63] CIP is the acronym for Congenital Insensitivity to Pain
[64] Luch A, ed. (2009). Molecular, clinical and
environmental toxicology. Springer. p. 20. ISBN 3-7643-
8335-6.
[65] NY Times, by Josh Katz, Sept 2, 2017
[66] IBID
[67] http://christianscience.com/what-is-christian-
science#relationship-with-western-medicine
[68] From the website, http://christianscience.com/what-
is-christian-science#relationship-with-western-medicine,
"over 80,000 Christian Science healings have been
published throughout the past 140 years, including
severe cases"
[69] A leper is a patient suffering from leprosy, primarily a
severely disfiguring disease of the poor, currently
affecting more than a quarter million people in the
world, mostly in India.
[70] Mucinous adenocarcinoma tumors are a type of cancer
that can start in the stomach, they account for about
10% of stomach cancers, and they are often highly
malignant.
[71] Jemal A, Bray F, Center MM, Ferlay J, Ward E, Forman
D, CA Cancer J Clin. 2011 Mar-Apr; 61(2):69-90.
[72] Research performed by Gopal K. Singh, a
demographer at the Department of Health and
Human Services, and Mohammad Siahpush, a
professor at the University of Nebraska Medical
Center in Omaha.
[73] Department of Health and Human services, Dr. Gopal
K. Singh, reported by New York Times:
http://www.nytimes.co
m/2008/03/23/us/23health.html?_r=0
[74] From a Merritt Hawkins study, 2014.
[75] Megan Macardle, The Atlantic, "How Much Does
Medicaid Improve Well-Being?" July 7, 2011

[76] Those in our population ranging in age from about 15 to 35, often with a self-perception of immortality.

[77] Health Insurance: Premiums and Increases, 10/30/2017, National Conference of State Legislatures.

[78] Alz.Org., http://www.alz.org/alzheimers_disease_steps_to_diagnosis.asp

[79] 25-30 % of the population would be positive since these patients already have this gene and most of them won't get Alzheimer's disease. As a positive test for a disease that isn't present or that won't develop, a very large number of these results could be considered false positives.

[80] CDC: http://www.cdc.gov/measles/cases-outbreaks.html

[81] NBC News: http://www.nbcnews.com/storyline/measles-outbreak/measles-outbreak-traced-disneyland-declared-over-n343686

[82] Melissa Pamer, KTLA Channel 5, http://ktla.com/2015/06/30/gov-brown-signs-law-ending-personal-religious-exemptions-to-school-vaccine-requirements/

[83] Also called a "concierge" practice by many, a term I have disliked because of the nobility implications.

[84] This retainer slowly increased *for new patients only* to $3,000 over the subsequent 13 years; the price of entry, however, stays the same throughout the patients' lifetimes.

[85] Apparently at the request of his father, Vernon Presley: http://biography.yourdictionary.com/articles/how-did-elvis-presley-die.html

[86] Reuters, August 28, 2009, http://www.reuters.com/article/us-jackson-idUSTRE57R4EY20090828

[87] Adam Higginbotham (August 11, 2002). "Elvis' special Doctor Feelgood". The Observer.

[88] 3/12/2014 12:55 AM PDT BY TMZ STAFF, http://www.tmz.com/2014/03/12/conrad-murray-michael-jackson-trinidad-doctor-practice-medicine/

[89] Associated press: http://www.usatoday.com/story/news/nation/2013/10/

28/jacksons-doctor-released/3284617/

[90] The Oath of Hippocrates, one of the oldest binding documents in history, is as applicable to doctors today as it was to the physicians of about 4,000 years ago. I had recited the oath upon graduation from medical school and I recalled the relevant portion in these circumstances: "Whatsoever house I may enter, my visit shall be for the convenience and advantage of the patient; and I will willingly refrain from doing any injury or wrong from falsehood, and particularly from acts of an amorous nature..."

[91] Transference can be manifested as an erotic attraction, or otherwise emotional feelings, towards a physician or other therapist, often a psychiatrist, who takes the place of somebody in the past; the previous feelings for others are then transferred to the therapist.

[92] A Latin phrase meaning "first, do no harm." Although this concept is referenced in the Hippocratic Oath, the specific wording of this statement is not contained within the oath.

[93] Per the California Health and Safety Code Section 1799.102; "No person who in good faith, and not for compensation, renders emergency medical or nonmedical care at the scene of an emergency shall be liable for any civil damages resulting from any act or omission." The law also clarifies that a person cannot be held liable for civil damages unless their actions or omissions constitute "gross negligence or willful or wanton misconduct. "

[94] His real name.

[95] Jack Dolan, Los Angeles Times, http://www.latimes.com/local/california/la-me-0829-doctor-convicted-20150829-story.html

[96] NY Times, Tuesday, February 9, 2016: http://www.nytimes.com/health/guides/disease/alcoholism/possible-complications.html

[97] NIH, National Institute of Alcohol abuse and Alcoholism, http://pubs.niaaa.nih.gov/publications/arh25-4/282-287.htm

[98] Alcoholics Anonymous: Alcoholics Anonymous is an international fellowship of men and women who have had a drinking problem. It is nonprofessional, self-

supporting, multiracial, apolitical, and available almost everywhere. There are no age or education requirements. Membership is open to anyone who wants to do something about his or her drinking problem. http://www.aa.org/pages/en_US/what-is-aa

[99]Gina Kolata and Sarah Cohen, Jan. 16, 2016, New York Times http://www.nytimes.com/2016/01/17/science/drug-overdoses-propel-rise-in-mortality-rates-of-young-whites.html?_r=0

[100] Geoff Taylor, Senior VP, Corporate Communications & Public Policy, https://www.health.ny.gov/health_care/medicaid/redesign/docs/2011-10-17_medical_malpractice_premiums.pdf

[101] Excellus, Mello MM, Chandra A, Gawande AA, Studdert DM: "National Costs of the Medical Liability System." Health Affairs, Vol. 29 , No. 9, pages 1569-1577. http://content.healthaffairs.org/content/29/9/1569.abstract or http://health.burgess.house.gov/UploadedFiles/Malpractice-Health_Affairs.pdf

[102] The most reliable measurement for diabetes (A1C) had not yet been invented.

[103]John Adams, Novanglus Essays, No. 7, produced in 1775. The "Novanglus" letters were a systematic attempt by Adams to describe the origins, nature, and jurisdictional boundaries of the imperial British constitution.

[104] POLST: Physician Orders for Life Sustaining Treatment-- The POLST Paradigm was developed to improve the quality of patient care and reduce medical errors by creating a system that identifies patients' wishes regarding medical treatment and communicates and respects them by creating portable medical orders the paramedics will follow. http://www.polst.org/about-the-national-polst-paradigm/what-is-polst/ . The actual form is at: https://www.cdph.ca.gov/programs/LnC/Documents/MDS30-ApprovedPOLSTForm.pdf

[105] The Death with Dignity form is at: http://www.doh.wa.gov/portals/1/Documents/Pubs/422-063-

RequestMedicationEndMyLifeHumaneDignifiedManner.p
df

[106] Described in detail at the POLST site:
http://www.polst.org/wp-
content/uploads/2015/11/2015.10.05-DWD-POLST-
Statement.pdf

[107] A summary of each state's requirements may be
found at:
http://www.caringinfo.org/i4a/pages/index.cfm?pageid=
3289

[108] Laurie A, Neimeyer RA, University of Memphis,
Tennessee, retrieved from:
http://www.ncbi.nlm.nih.gov/pubmed/18680889.

[109] Grief Speaks: Culture and Grief, retrieved from:
http://www.griefspeaks.com/id90.html.

[110] Hines Smith, 2002, Death Studies, 26, 309-323.

[111] The term black church or African-American church
often refers to Protestant Christian churches that have
ministered to predominantly black congregations in the
United States.

[112] Neighbors, Harold; Musick, Marc; Williams, David
(1998). "The African American Minister as a Source of
Help for Serious Personal Crises"

[113] the cycle of death and rebirth with which life in the
material world is bound

[114] Everplans: Buddhist funeral traditions, extracted from
https://www.everplans.com/articles/buddhist-funeral-
traditions

[115] JTB, retrieved from:
http://www.japanspecialist.co.uk/travel-tips/shinto-
buddhism/

[116]https://en.wikipedia.org/wiki/History_of_immigration
_to_the_United_States

[117] Sepsis refers to the presence of harmful bacteria and
their toxins in tissues.

[118] Background review may be recovered from:
http://www.oie.int/doc/ged/D12405.PDF

[119] 70-80% prevention by vaccination. Recovered from:
https://www.aphis.usda.gov/animal_health/animal_dise
ases/brucellosis/downloads/bruc-facts.pdf

[120] Brucellosis may be caused by local animals producing
milk which, if not pasteurized, is known as "raw milk" but
vaccination has greatly reduced the incident of the

disease: In 1956, there were 124,000 affected herds found by testing in the United States. By 1992, this number had dropped to 700 herds and the number of affected, domestic herds has declined to single digits since then, extracted from: https://www.aphis.usda.gov/animal_health/animal_dise ases/brucellosis/downloads/bruc-facts.pdf

[121] Beyond Words: WHAT ANIMALS THINK AND FEEL, Henry Holt and Company, LLC. July, 2015.

[122] http://www.gorongosa.org/our-story/our-team/joyce-poole

[123] Carolyn Y. Johnson, Globe Staff , 7/11/12, Native Americans migrated to the New World in three waves, Harvard-led DNA analysis shows, recovered from: Boston.com, http://www.boston.com/whitecoatnotes/2012/07/11/na tive-americans-migrated-the-new-world-three-waves-harvard-led-dna-analysis-shows/uQRQdkkqMmzSW3LaArh0tM/story.html

[124] Now off the market and sold as mefloquin.

[125] There are approximately 3,500 different species of mosquitoes, grouped into 41 different groups, each called a genus. Of these groups, only one—*Anopheles*—can carry and transmit malaria (from: http://www.cdc.gov/malaria/about/biology/ mosquitoes/ ).

[126] Naturally acquired immunity to the parasite known as Plasmodium falciparum.

[127] Extracted from: https://www.againstmalaria.com/downloads/RBMBurde nMalariaAfrica.pdf

[128] There has already been a 60% reduction in worldwide mortality since the year 2000 (from WHO: http://www.who.int/features/factfiles/malaria/en/ ) mostly because of insect eradication.

[129] The Kavli Prize, awarded every two years by the Kavli Foundation, initiated by the late Fred Kavli in 2008, to honor and support scientists whose work is considered to be exceptionally exciting in the 21st Century in the fields of astrophysics, nanoscience, and neuroscience.

[130] Research performed by Dr. Cornelia Isabella "Cori" Bargmann , an American neurobiologist, known for her work on the behavior in the C. elegans, particularly

olfaction in the worm.

[131] Retrieved from:
https://www.google.com/webhp?sourceid=chrome-instant&ion=1&espv=2&ie=UTF-8#q=human%20brain%20number%20of%20neurons

[132] Heidi Godman, Executive Editor, *Harvard Health Letter,* retrieved from
http://www.health.harvard.edu/blog/regular-exercise-changes-brain-improve-memory-thinking-skills-201404097110

[133]http://www.nytimes.com/health/guides/symptoms/depression/print.html

[134] To be presented at: American Academy of Neurology's 68th Annual Meeting in Vancouver, Canada, April 15 to 21, 2016, retrieved from:
https://www.aan.com/PressRoom/Home/PressRelease/1440

[135] King's College London. "Depression as deadly as smoking, study finds." ScienceDaily. ScienceDaily, 18 November 2009.

[136] An Inflammatory Theory of Brain Disease, by Lauren Aguirre on Wed, 25 Feb 2015, retrieved from:
http://www.pbs.org/wgbh/nova/next/body/brain-inflammation/

[137] Aortic Dissection, John W. Hallett, Jr., MD

[138] Aortic Dissection, Frank J. Criado, MD, FACS, Joseph S. Coselli, MD, Section Editor, U.S. National Library of Medicine, NIH (National Institutes of Health) retrieved from:http://www.ncbi.nlm.nih.gov/pmc/articles/PMC3233335/

Made in the USA
San Bernardino, CA
20 February 2018